P

THE MENO

Caroline Hawkridge did her postgraduate training in health education after receiving a BSc in Psychology and Physiology. She worked for eight years in the National Health Service, ran a training project for the Health Education Council/National Extension College and has taught several health courses for the Open University.

Caroline Hawkridge wrote the first British book on endometriosis, then a little-known gynaecological condition, having co-founded the women's health charity the Endometriosis Society (1981–9). *Understanding Endometriosis* (1989) received widespread publicity and was well reviewed in the *Lancet*, *New Scientist* and *Nursing Times*. It is now in its second edition as *Living with Endometriosis* (1996). She has also written the endometriosis section in the second edition of *Our Bodies, Ourselves* (Penguin, 1991) and co-authored a chapter in *Disorders of the Menstrual Cycle* (1988).

She now writes full-time. She has appeared on national television, radio and in the press, most recently on the subject of young women on HRT. She wrote this book after her own early menopause.

The Menopause, HRT and You

CAROLINE HAWKRIDGE

PENGUIN BOOKS

This book is not intended as a substitute for medical advice from a qualified doctor or health professional and shouldn't be used as such. Every effort has been made by the author and publisher to ensure that the information given is correct at the time of publication. However, research is very active in this area and it is possible that new data will supersede the findings presented here.

PENGUIN BOOKS

Published by the Penguin Group
Penguin Books Ltd, 27 Wrights Lane, London w8 5tz, England
Penguin Putnam Inc., 375 Hudson Street, New York, New York 10014, USA
Penguin Books Australia Ltd, Ringwood, Victoria, Australia
Penguin Books Canada Ltd, 10 Alcorn Avenue, Toronto, Ontario, Canada m4v 3b2
Penguin Books (NZ) Ltd, Private Bag 102902, NSMC, Auckland, New Zealand

Penguin Books Ltd, Registered Offices: Harmondsworth, Middlesex, England

Published in 1999
1 3 5 7 9 10 8 6 4 2

Set in 10/13pt Monotype Sabon
Typeset by Rowland Phototypesetting Ltd,
Bury St Edmunds, Suffolk
Printed in England by Clays Ltd, St Ives plc

For Graham, and the children in my life,
Catherine, Rachel, Tegan and Michael.

CONTENTS

ACKNOWLEDGEMENTS

My special thanks go to the support groups who allowed me to share and learn, the Androgen Insensitivity Syndrome (AIS) Support Group, UK Turner Society, Premature Menopause Support Group, Ovacome and the Child Growth Foundation. It has been a pleasure.

A lot of people made this book possible by trusting, telling, writing, listening, reading, e-mailing, passing me on, musing, pondering, scribbling, editing, illustrating, laughing, suggesting and believing: Alan, Antonia, Audrey, Bungy, Clair, Doreen, Eileen, Emma, Frances, Ingrid, Juanita, Julia, Kate, Rachel, Rosemary, Rosie, Susan, Joanne Austin, Jane Baldwin, Felicity Bates, Maureen Bradley, Juliet Burton, Dr Gerard Conway, Catherine Corp, Mary Davis, Claire Duchen, Waltraud L. Field, Monique Francis, Vreli Fry, Betty Gadsby, David Gifford, Denise Goddard, Eleo Gordon, Sherri Groveman, Mr Sean Hughes, Dr Susan Kagan-Krieger, Andrea Lacey, Lynnette Lowes, Alison Lyon, Mr Keith Masters, Diane Mathews, Angela Merry, Angela Miles, Kathy Mill, Jennifer Milligan, Pip and Brian Morris, Pippa Ogier, Claire Péligry, J. E. Price, Teresa Pugh, Josephine Roe, Andrea Shield, Val Stagg, Rachel and Kate Thould, Alexandra Whates, Lisa Whiting and Janet Woolmer. Several people did not wish to be named but their assistance has been very welcome.

I also wish to acknowledge the Turner's Syndrome Society of the US, Victorian Turner's Syndrome Association Inc. (Australia), Premature Ovarian Failure Support Group (USA), Bank St Writers, Crewe and District Writers' Circle, Forum Writers (Wythenshawe) and Women's Institute (Cheshire), and thank the Premature Menopause Support Group (formerly Daisy Chain) for permission to update Pip's and Brian's stories.

Finally I am grateful to my family and friends at home and abroad. Every little helped.

FOREWORD

By Dr Gerard S. Conway
Consultant Endocrinologist, The Middlesex Hospital, London
Honorary Senior Lecturer, University College, London

The twentieth century has brought many changes to the lives of women. Among these, one has proved to be of increasing concern – the menopause. For the first time in history, life expectancy for the majority of women extends beyond reproductive life. Thus we are the only species in which a menopause has a major impact. How are menopausal women supposed to consider this situation? Is the menopause a natural event that should not be tampered with? Or is it an artificial consequence of improved living conditions? Caught in this conundrum, many women find it difficult to obtain informed answers to their questions. In this volume, many of them will find the insight into the menopause that they were unable to find elsewhere.

In the ideal world a woman entering the menopause who wishes to evaluate for herself the pros and cons of HRT would be able to call upon the expertise of several specialists. An epidemiologist to interpret the large studies of the risks and benefits of HRT, a gynae-cologist to evaluate the physical effects of oestrogen deficiency, a psychologist to guide her through this information in perspective of other life events, a pharmacologist to guide her through the maze of different preparations, and an alternative practitioner or two to present the merits of their approach. In the real world one would be lucky to meet even one of these specialists. In the following pages we find that the contribution from each of these specialities is presented with the user in mind so that every reader can find a balance of opinion.

While it may have been difficult for women who are approaching the average age of the menopause to find informed advice, the prospect for women entering an early menopause has been hopeless. This is a key area that has been opened up for the first time in this book. The issues concerning women experiencing the menopause in their teens, twenties or thirties have long been neglected. Specialists, frustrated at being able to offer no insight into the cause of early ovarian failure and little in the way of fertility treatment, have tended to leave women floundering alone. We now realize that early ovarian failure carries major psychological and physical consequences. Psychological support is rarely made available to young women who confront early permanent infertility at a time when they might be just coming to terms with their sexuality. The social isolation that follows the diagnosis of premature ovarian failure in this age group can affect relationships throughout life. An early menopause, after all, does not fall easily into teenage conversation.

For similar reasons, any disorder of sexual development diagnosed in young life is extraordinarily difficult to cope with. Over the past 10 years a period of enlightenment has taken place for women with intersex disorders such as androgen insensitivity. The difficulties of coming to terms with an intersex diagnosis and the inhibitions surrounding the subject are clearly brought out in Chapter 6. The personal experiences made available here will go a long way to make others feel less alone with their condition and to compensate for the limited support available through the health service. Any doctor working in the field will learn a lot from these accounts, particularly regarding the confusion that their profession often inadvertently leaves in its wake.

With regard to HRT, we are only beginning to understand that the concerns for young women may differ from those commonly discussed for older women. Have we got the dose of oestrogen optimized for safe use over 40 years? How should we best monitor such long-term use? It would be too much to expect any book to have all the answers to these questions – they simply do not exist. By raising the collective awareness of this subject, however, this book will enable women to ask more searching questions in their medical consultations – the more difficult the better. It is only in this way that we in the medical professions will be motivated to collect the data required to inform the next generation with the detail they have a right to expect.

On a practical level, all women will learn the pros and cons of various forms of HRT. With more than 50 preparations on the market, an independent guide through the maze is sorely needed. Also, the frustration of finding a suitable and tolerable form of HRT finds a rarely heard voice here in several contributions. Many women will be pleased to discover that others find that HRT is no panacea.

For all these reasons this book is warmly welcomed. It will offer reassurance to many and stimulate discussion for all.

I

EIGHT WOMEN

For Eileen it was all over during a shopping trip. Josephine just had to 'get on with it' and Audrey is still wondering how to cope. Kate tried hormone replacement therapy (HRT).

One way or another, most women will go through the natural menopause. However, some women have the menopause unexpectedly early, perhaps due to surgery or cancer treatment, or for unknown reasons. Jane was 34 when her ovaries were removed. Pip was 16 when her periods began – and ended. Both were prescribed hormone replacement therapy.

Other women need HRT from an early age due to genetic conditions. Bungy was born without functioning ovaries and eventually discovered that she had Turner syndrome. Rosemary knew something was wrong, but she spent 31 years on HRT before learning that she had a rare intersex condition. Both these women had very disturbing experiences due to a lack of medical understanding.

In this chapter, women of all ages begin to talk about what the menopause and the question of HRT has meant for them. Their stories are not intended to be representative; instead, they raise some of the dilemmas explored in this book.

Eileen's Story

My menopause happened when I was about 44. At the time I was busy and happy – as I have been for most of my life.

My youngest child was six years old and the other three were aged up to 17. My periods had been becoming irregular and slight and then, one day when I was in town, I had a mighty and unexpected bleed. My thoughts were about the difficulties of the situation – I suffered not at all! Except for a few times when I was in my twenties and living abroad, away from home and friends, I have not really experienced period pains.

I was glad to have passed the menopause and, after a time, to be free to abandon birth control while continuing an active sex life – rather better than in the last years before the menopause. I have never felt the need for exploring HRT (perhaps because my general health has been good all my life and I have been blessed with much happiness). There has always been plenty to do outside the home. I think I have been influenced, subconsciously, by the Bible teaching of 'Freely you have received, freely give'. Most of my work, in and out of the family, has been a pleasure. All that sounds rather dull and undramatic – and all of *that* sounds hopelessly SMUG! I am so aware of the difficulties that many women experience, and osteoporosis may be important for all.

Josephine's Story

I was 15 when I had my first period and 49 years old when I had my last. I went through the menopause from the age of 40 onwards but, when I was 47, I found myself homeless because of divorce. So, due to circumstances, I obtained 'living-in' jobs in hotels, which meant I worked hard and had no time to dwell on my age. Mind over matter, so to speak. My five children had grown up by then.

My last two periods were the worst I had ever had, both were very heavy and lasted three to four weeks. After that – nothing. In order to avoid being 'washed out' I had a Guinness every night before retiring, which I think helped me overcome tiredness and lack of energy. HRT was never mentioned then and I rarely saw a doctor. My mother's advice to me was, 'The menopause is a natural occurrence, therefore keep yourself busy and "get on with it".'

I am now aged 73 and, from the age of 52, I have been on alternative medicine – selenium, zinc, oil of evening primrose, kelp and calcium – and I also bath with sea-salt crystals. I feel they are expensive, but in order to afford them, I buy food which is cheap but nutritional. My diet has always been porridge oats, rice and pasta, greens, all fruit, black strap molasses, garlic, tuna, barley, etc. I feel fine. However, I think HRT is very beneficial to most women; three of my daughters have it and they are 'blooming'.

Audrey's Story

I am 47 and just now I don't really know whether I am coming or going! I had the occasional hot flush at first, but didn't think much of it. I would get a bit too warm but things weren't bad, I thought. Then I didn't come on period-wise for about four months. That's when I started with what I call the 'hot clammy' kind.

Before one started, I would feel odd, like I was about to remember that I'd forgotten something and, next thing, this heat was rushing to my face. There's nothing you can do. No one seemed to notice at work, which is something, I suppose, but you don't know if everyone is being polite. I felt like a lighthouse! Next to that, the worst is when sweat trickles down your front and your hair sticks to your scalp, also down your neck. Sometimes it is a wonder that my glasses don't steam up!

Luckily I can always find an excuse to get out of the office to the ladies' toilet and freshen up. Sometimes I feel better just for running my wrists under the cold tap; I can always pretend I'm washing my hands if someone comes in. I'm glad I'm not with the girls behind the counter in front of customers. Being behind that glass would give me flushes, I'm sure, and then what can you do? Being in the lift at work can start me off, especially if it's a squeeze. I'm only one floor up, so I use the stairs and nowadays you can laugh that off as a health thing. I dare say the exercise is good for me.

The sweating at night has been difficult because my husband travels a lot and often gets a really early train. Sometimes I wake him with throwing off the covers. Then I might be getting back to sleep and his alarm will go; neither of us can win. At least our youngest daughter, the only one at home now, is 15 and old enough to sort herself most mornings, because some days I don't do anything straight.

I tried milk drinks and those 'sleeptime' tea-bags but I was up in the night for the toilet, so I got some herbal tablets from the chemist. They had valerian in them and you could take two to four so I tried two, but even four didn't do much. I tried a different sort from the health-food shop. They helped a bit, but made me foggy next morning, which was almost as bad as when I wasn't sleeping. Being exhausted at the end of the day doesn't seem to make any difference; I still wake up sweaty and clammy. Always sometime after midnight, maybe because it is a hormonal thing. Sometimes lately I go downstairs and watch videos. It feels better than lying awake, although the dog must wonder what I'm about!

Since this started, the menopause, my periods have been off and on. When they came back on, after stopping the first time, the hot flushes disappeared and I got some sleep! Except one period carried on for two weeks, which was beginning to worry me. Now I've started missing again, the flushes and sweats are back. I think this is how it's going to be but, there again, you don't really know. I would say I am coping, but I am not sure how long all this is going to go on for. The tiredness is the hardest part because I don't want people at work to think I'm getting absent-minded in my old age or have worries at home. I don't want to go to my doctor because I don't hold with taking anything strong.

Kate's Story

I am 55 years of age; I suppose I started experiencing problems around the age 40, three years after the birth of our youngest son, but really didn't take too much notice. My hair was thinning and my skin was getting very dry, but the most worrying problem for me was memory loss and lack of coordination. Even my speech was affected insofar as sentences came out back to front. I was also unnaturally tired even after a good night's sleep. I put up with this for years. It was only after collapsing that I finally visited my GP. After various blood tests, a hormonal but not menopausal imbalance was diagnosed and I started taking HRT tablets. At that stage, I was happy to take anything to relieve my terrible fatigue.

Within a few months I started getting severe headaches; there was no regular pattern but any small thing would trigger them – a short car ride with the air directed on my head, a room full of noise, getting too tired, numerous things. I told my GP when I was called in for the regular six-monthly HRT check-up. My prescription was changed quite a few times over the next six years. I remember trying Estracombi skin patches, but the migraine was becoming more regular, twice a month, and lasting three days. I said I couldn't continue but tried, as a last resort, the new Kliofem (2 mg tablets), but this too was unsuccessful.

I decided to stop taking HRT three years ago. I increased my daily dose of evening primrose oil from 500 mg to 1000 mg and also took a multi-vitamin and mineral supplement. I felt absolutely fine, experienced no withdrawal symptoms and only very occasionally now get a headache. I have not had a period or any menopausal symptoms, such as hot flushes, since.

I had a bone density scan five months ago, after getting pain in my neck and noticing a lump at the top of my spine. My mother and grandmother both suffered from osteoarthritis. This scan showed a low bone density and I have started taking Fosamax (alendronate sodium 10 mg). I will now be scanned every two years. I have not been told how long I will be on Fosamax, but I got the impression that it would be a long time and I am not too happy about that. Fosamax is not easy to take. I have to swallow it with half a pint of water immediately on waking and then wait half an hour before taking food and drink. I cannot bend or lie down until I have eaten as this causes burning in the oesophagus and throat. There was no information available from my GP so I had to ask around various friends, one of whom is a pharmacist, and through her I obtained the write-up on Fosamax, which I found most helpful.

I have found all the way along this road that I would have liked more information on the drugs I was being asked to take. I like to know what I am taking, how it works in my body and what side-effects it may cause – I need to feel happy with it. I feel that this information should have been available from my GP; it is out there but one has to know where to look.

Jane's Story

I had a hysterectomy and removal of ovaries in September last year, aged 34.

I had suspected for some time that I was suffering from endometriosis because of the increasing pain during menstruation. Although my periods had never been easy – I started aged ten – they had never been so debilitating and analgesics were not touching the pain at all. Because of my past training as a nurse I knew that the only way to diagnose was with an exploratory op (laparoscopy) and so I kept putting off consulting my GP. However, one night I woke up with pain which became so acute that I vomited. My husband, who had spent many a night up with me by this stage, insisted that I do something about it.

Within two weeks endometriosis was confirmed with a laparoscopy. Apparently the vomiting was the result of a so-called 'chocolate' [dark brown blood-filled] cyst bursting on the ovary. The endometriosis was very severe. Both ovaries were affected and the Fallopian tubes had thickened and twisted back on themselves causing one ovary to stick to the wall of the uterus. I also had multiple large fibroids. Within another two weeks I had had the hysterectomy. I was started on oral oestrogen four days later.

The aftercare was basically non-existent. I saw my consultant again after six weeks, but little advice was offered as to the emotional effects, which I found surprising considering I was relatively young, childless and had a history of anxiety and mild depression in my late twenties. When I asked my GP surgery for details of support groups or information for women after hysterectomy, I was told to contact a Citizens Advice Bureau!

It took some time for me to adjust to the HRT. Initially I was given Progynova 2 mg tablets, but four months later, when I asked for a blood test to check my hormone levels as I was feeling tired and 'low', it showed that I was in effect experiencing the menopause as my body had not absorbed the hormone in tablet form. The blood test also showed that my testosterone levels were extremely high as I had had a testosterone implant during surgery (as my gynaecologist felt it had some efficacy in treating post-operative tiredness and loss of libido). But instead of releasing the normal female amounts the implant was releasing too much. It was to be replaced every eight months for three years or more but I decided against replacement. In my opinion, it had no real benefit.

I was put on Estraderm 100 patches, but, again, there were problems with absorption as they came off easily in the bath and would 'rumple up' quite often. I was then put on Estraderm Mx100, which is different in design and sticks much better. So far blood tests show that I am now obtaining enough oestrogen [see page 60].

During this time I changed doctors within the surgery. This is because when I visited my GP about the difficulty with my first patches, his response to my tearfulness and tiredness was to prescribe antidepressants. I did not take these. What was required was simply careful monitoring of the HRT. It is so important to have a GP one can trust and who will monitor the treatment properly.

Obviously, as I am only in my thirties, it has been important for me to get plenty of oestrogen so I would not take only herbal alternatives. However, I do use essential oils, such as clary sage, which have a similar molecular structure to natural oestrogens [see Figure 4.2, page 62]. I also eat quite a lot of soya, which has similar properties.

Interestingly, my feet indicated for years that I had gynaecological problems. I am a reflexologist, but whilst having treatment on my own feet I learned they were always sensitive in the regions to do with reproduction. Since the hysterectomy my feet have told a different story.

I have put on a considerable amount of weight since the operation, although my diet is the same – I am a vegetarian. I have gone up almost two dress sizes. Although my husband has been extremely supportive about this, I had quite a bit of difficulty in adjusting to my altered body image.

Complicating all of this is the fact that I was beginning to think seriously about the possibility of having children. Although neither of us had felt that children were necessary to our happiness, at 34 I was not as sure as I had been in the past. For me, the problems of recovery and adjustment were exacerbated by feelings of intense regret – which I have still. At 22 I had a termination of a pregnancy and so my thoughts were peppered with 'what ifs', as well as a sense that I was being justly punished. The decision to have the termination was not easy.

I completely agree with my husband that we should enjoy life for what it is and, as we are here for such a short time, we should make the most of it. And yet, for me, the main problem has been a sense of having been cut adrift from life's cycle. Paradoxically I miss my 'moon monthlies' (as periods were often described in the past), however painful they may have been.

I had always felt sorry for men because they were not so overtly connected with the rhythms of Nature. The internal photographs of my ovaries and womb taken during the laparoscopy showed something resembling planets in orbit – a universe in microcosm. With their removal I have felt at times empty in more senses than one, no longer a part of the great scheme of things.

To end on an optimistic note, it is good not to suffer the dreaded PMT any longer and my husband seconds that. Also I am no longer prone to anaemia or asthma, which I had suffered since childhood. And of course to be free of the severe pain of endometriosis has been liberating. Sexually there have been no lasting problems although I do feel that orgasm is less intense. The future is obviously as yet an unknown entity for those of us on HRT from an early age, but I try not to dwell on this too much and, as the alternative is unacceptable to me, I just carry on.

Pip and Brian's Story

Pip

Aged 16, I had three periods over one year. No more came and every time my mother took me to the GP she was told to come back in three months' time, that things would probably settle down and that there was nothing wrong with me.

I did feel different from other girls – I was never into make-up, fashion, discos, etc., and I found it very hard to relate to boys. I was never a typical teenager and didn't rebel at all. I became a private, introverted person who found it hard to talk and I was becoming confused and afraid about why my periods didn't come.

I felt a freak and found it hard when my girlfriends talked about their boyfriends and going on the Pill. I used to be very embarrassed about the whole issue. I had even done childcare at school and, according to the teacher, there was never a problem with infertility and 'an egg is produced every month'. Why wasn't this happening to me?

By 20, my GP (who virtually laughed at me when I said I didn't feel normal) at last referred me to a gynaecologist. After various tests he told me in a matter-of-fact manner that my ovaries didn't work, he didn't know why and they probably wouldn't work in the future. I'd have to take HRT for the rest of my life and I'd never have children. What HRT was for or why I had to take it wasn't explained.

To be honest, it didn't mean much to me then, probably because when I had my regular 'bleed' on HRT I felt more normal and part of the gang. Also I was heavily into ponies and was never going to get married, let alone have children! The whole thing was kept secret and very few people knew about it.

I went on to Prempak-C at 22 and very quickly became bloated, putting on a lot of weight. This was so hard. People teased me about my size and I was so embarrassed by it all – I knew it wasn't from overeating but I couldn't tell the truth. I later changed to Trisequens, which seemed to suit me.

I met Brian when I was 23. We were serious about each other from the start and I knew I was going to have to tell him. It was very hard – I hadn't known him long and I didn't feel he'd stick around; also I'd never had to tell anyone before. He was brilliant. Instead of running away, he just hugged me and said it didn't bother him and he loved me for who I was. I couldn't believe this. To me, it ruled my life. What a failure I was. I wasn't even a woman, I couldn't even give him a child (which after all is what women are here for, or so I believed at the time). Something as simple as producing an egg, what every woman could do, and I couldn't.

We got engaged quickly and then the next people to tell were his parents – made even more difficult by the fact that Brian is an only child. Then I contracted ME [myalgic encephalomyelitis]. It was awful. On top of everything else, I now became frustrated and angry at what I couldn't do physically. It stopped me horse-riding and doing any sports.

As soon as we were married, the comments began: 'When are you starting a family, then?' I found it so hard; people just treated it as one big joke. I became depressed and Brian persuaded me to see a counsellor; he couldn't take the pressure any more. Talking to someone really eased the burden enormously. She helped me to see that it wasn't my fault and boosted my self-confidence greatly. She also gave us the courage to tell people. We couldn't believe how understanding our friends and relatives were.

Two and a half years after getting married and being on a waiting list for egg-donation IVF, we had our first appointment. It was only then that I found out exactly what had happened to me. When I had my three periods, instead of them starting puberty, they were in fact the end. When I was in the womb, I had developed normally and my ovaries and eggs were all present and correct. However, the 'time-clock' relating to them had been triggered (by what, they don't know), and even before I was born, my eggs were being used up. So by the time I was 17 all my eggs had gone. It was so much easier having an explanation. I didn't feel so much of a freak now that I knew I had had some eggs.

Our treatment went ahead quickly and we were so lucky because it worked first time. I gave up work and enjoyed my pregnancy and ever-expanding tummy. About this time I heard about the Premature Menopause Support Group. It has helped me enormously to talk to other women who have experienced premature menopause. I thought I was the only one in the whole wide world!

When our beautiful son was born, it was such a special, magical moment. I never thought I'd ever give birth.

I breastfed for a year, so didn't take any HRT, and then a strange thing happened – I started having regular monthly bleeds! My GP did tests: I wasn't ovulating but my hormone levels had risen enough to induce bleeding. We had two unsuccessful attempts at egg-donation IVF and then, a year after my first bleed, my GP discovered I *was* ovulating! We got in touch with our IVF clinic immediately (as they had an egg donor ready). They were as amazed as we were and said I'd been wrongly diagnosed and had had resistant ovary syndrome (everything *is* there but it wasn't working, although, again, we don't know why). What a shock!

We arranged to see the consultant to find out more, but then had to cancel two days beforehand because I was pregnant! The terrible thing is that I had a miscarriage, which we are still trying to come to terms with, as well as the wrong diagnosis *and* a pregnancy. There is so much uncertainty because we don't know if I'll ever have periods again.

Brian

Pip and I met eight years ago. Within a few weeks of our meeting, she told me she couldn't have children. It didn't bother me at all; I hadn't really thought about marriage and children as such, but probably I would have wanted children in time. It didn't change the way I felt about Pip, even though she found that very hard to understand. She thought I'd leave and never come back after she told me about her premature menopause. It was so hard watching her cry night after night – I felt so hopeless and helpless – there was nothing I could do. To me it was just one aspect of her life that wasn't really a problem. To her it was one huge part of her life that *was* a problem.

We were married in our mid twenties and only our parents knew about our situation. We went on to the egg-donation IVF list immediately. We were told we'd have to wait a long time, but didn't feel this would be too much of a problem. After two and a half years it was! Friends kept asking us, 'When are you going to have children?' and 'About time you had kids, isn't it?'

It got harder. First we laughed it off, then it got to both of us. What was really difficult for me was seeing Pip getting more upset, frustrated and depressed as time went on. I dreaded telling her about friends who were getting pregnant, even more so if it was an 'accident' or even a 'mistake'. I became very worried and persuaded her to see a counsellor. I just couldn't take the pressure and I didn't know the answers to her questions, like 'Why?' and 'Why me?' I supported her as much as I could, though we very nearly split up over the stress we were under. It was a very hard time, but one thing that really helped us was deciding to go public and tell friends and relatives – that took a huge amount of pressure off.

We finally got our first appointment for IVF. What a sense of achievement! I was excited that it was happening, but worried about Pip and the possible consequences. We weren't prepared for all the questions we had to face to be realistic about our chances. In two months they'd found an egg donor that matched and the whole treatment began. One week before fertilization day I developed an infection in my sperm and had to take penicillin. Luckily it cleared up and everything went ahead. Having to produce a sperm sample on the day was nerve-wracking because so much depended on me. Three days later, two embryos were implanted into Pip. I held her hand and prayed.

The next two weeks were the longest in my life. I went from feeling pessimistic to optimistic and back again. I felt Pip was far too hopeful and was worried about how to cope if the pregnancy test was negative. The first pregnancy test didn't work. We couldn't believe it. The second one came up with a very faint positive, so I went straight out and bought two more. It was the happiest day of my life – Pip was pregnant!

Lots of tears and hugs. I don't really think it hit either of us, though it was a dream come true. We told our friends and relatives straight away – we felt that they'd been so supportive before that we wanted them to share our wonderful news. Pip's pregnancy went well. I was present at the birth and I wouldn't have missed it for the world. Our special son weighed in at 10 lb! There were tears and hugs. An absolute dream come true.

Bungy's Story

I was born in 1946. To begin with, I had some oedema [swelling] of face, feet and hands. On first sight, my Godmothers gave me the nickname Bungy, which family and friends still use! Little did my Godmothers know that they had picked up on an early diagnosis of Turner syndrome (TS) [see Chapter 6].

I had an infection at three weeks old (possibly the urinary tract), also common with Turner syndrome, and was one of the early post-war babies in the Midlands to be treated with antibiotics. But nothing was said on any diagnosis of Turner syndrome.

My mother, in particular, had concerns about my lack of growth, as I did, as I was not growing as much as my elder sister and two younger brothers. Puberty did not occur for me. I was seen by a GP who referred me to an endocrinologist. Being the late 1950s, C. E. Ford had just discovered the chromosome problem in Turner syndrome. I was admitted to hospital for a week of tests. My chromosome test had to be sent to London and Turner syndrome was confirmed.

The whole week was not a pleasant experience. I was frightened, confused and nobody told me what was happening. I did not ask and nobody said I had Turner syndrome. Although I was seen by a gynaecologist shortly afterwards, nothing further was done and I did not ask for anything more. I received no medication, no doctor suggested anything for me.

After boarding school, I trained as a nursery nurse, then I went into midwifery. Following this training, I went into a midwife-led general practitioner unit in a rural area, where I became a midwifery sister.

When I was 40, I received an invitation for a cervical smear, through my GP's computer system. I visited him and said I'd never had a cervical smear. He went through my notes. That was when I learnt I had Turner syndrome. He realized this was news to me and after that the practice, particularly a lady GP, were extremely kind and helpful.

I felt numb, angry and confused. By then, due to no medication, I had already developed osteoporosis, but it did not prevent me from work at that point. I was gradually introduced to hormones, which to my body felt totally strange. I had, of course, learnt about the feelings experienced by other women, if not myself, particularly as a midwife. I actually felt that for a year or two, psychologically, I needed to have 'periods' and have sanitary pads. Although somehow I felt embarrassed when they went through the supermarket check-out.

Although the osteoporosis improved on Prempak-C, I was having mood changes and after a year or so I found them difficult to cope with. I was also developing diabetes. There had been a latency for this which was exacerbated by stress. My father had a severe stroke in May 1987 and the GP unit where I worked was closed that Autumn, so I started working at a busy consultant unit. My gynaecologist transferred my hormone replacement to a then relatively new medication called Livial. He thought that at nearly 50 I would not wish to have periods any longer. This to me was marvellous. I have been taking Livial ever since, and my osteoporosis has been maintained at a satisfactory level, using Didronel and calcium also. However, because of my diabetes and the osteoporosis I retired at 44, now eight years ago.

I was extremely lucky to have a clinical psychologist, whom I had known while practising as a midwife, to go to talk to and express my feelings. The situation may well have been different without somebody to listen and, being a professional, guide me. There were a lot of feelings, particularly anger, to express. The hormone replacement helped me to feel a woman, but it was a great loss to me not to continue in my profession. As a midwifery sister, I was able to be with women at such an important time in their and their partner's life, and although I had not been able to have children myself, I was helping to bring new life into the world.

But I still have contact with some of my babies and their parents, and even met a mum through the Child Growth Foundation who recognized me after 12 years! She said I had delivered her daughter, who was diagnosed with Turner syndrome soon after birth. I had referred her from our unit to a paediatrician, but didn't know the diagnosis until her mother told me years later. Her daughter is now a teenager and doing well. She had growth hormone as a child and is now on hormone therapy. We have continued to meet up since then, and this has meant a lot to me.

This is where the big difference is with early diagnosis, correct treatment and full knowledge, so that the child grows up with that knowledge, compared to those days 30–40 years ago when little or no information and little or no treatment was given. These improvements help to satisfy me, and the fact the Society for Turner's Syndrome is there for the support and concern of parents, children and women. For me, meeting up with other women with Turner syndrome is now a vital part of my life.

Rosemary's Story

My happy childhood was followed by a troubled puberty. Eventually I was diagnosed as having a rare intersex condition known as androgen insensitivity syndrome (AIS) [see Chapter 6].

Aged 13–14: discovered, using a hand mirror, that something was not normal about my genitalia. I had lumps moving in my groin and no obvious vaginal opening. As I was an only child there was no one I could talk to, as this was not a subject one could broach with one's parents, so I kept this awful secret to myself.

15–17: travelled the world as a sportswoman. My mother kept packing sanitary towels in my luggage in case 'travelling brought it [menstruation] on', which of course it did not.

17+: my mother took me to our doctor who referred me to a London hospital. My initial examination was extremely frightening and embarrassing – my first contact was with a young male doctor. Over the next three months many tests were conducted – blood, a month's worth of urine, X-rays, naked photographs, culminating in an exploratory operation – the possible extent of which was never explained.

I awoke from this operation in a great deal of pain, not knowing what had happened. My parents were asked into an office. At the same time I was told hernias had been removed, there had been a problem in the development of my reproductive organs, and I could not have children. Also, I would need tablets for the rest of my life. My parents were told much the same story.

18–19: the oestrogen tablets (ethinyl oestradiol) greatly improved my appearance. I developed breasts and my complexion became 'fair' (almost transparent). I felt relieved that some progress had been made and started to live a more sociable life, as previously I had felt extremely stigmatized by my own feelings of not being normal.

I visited the hospital at regular intervals. More photographs were taken, but no information was forthcoming about my condition or treatment, nor was there any kind of counselling. The oestrogen tablets were dispensed annually by the gynaecologist. This arrangement continued for 28 years, even after she moved.

19–20: I met a young man and, when the question of sex arose, I told him what I knew of my condition. We embarked on a sexual relationship and during a hospital visit I mentioned this and was told an operation to create a vagina could only be carried out if marriage was likely. We were engaged and I entered hospital on my 21st birthday.

A diagram was drawn for me, and I underwent a Williams procedure. This was a very uncomfortable three weeks. After the wounds had healed, I was taught some pelvic-floor exercises and issued with a set of glass vaginal dilators. I attended clinics regularly. We got married six months later, and the Williams procedure was a qualified success.

22–23: saw a newspaper article headlined 'Female Athlete Had Hidden Testicles' and this struck a chord. Went to GP on another matter and asked about my case. He looked in my notes and said casually, 'You have XY chromosomes.' End of conversation. This piece of information was branded into my mind.

30–32: marriage fails for various reasons.

32–34: new relationship and marriage. At 39, I was invited to a conference hosted by my gynaecologist. I was kept outside until the end, when I was ushered in and seated on a 'stage' to answer questions from the floor, including 'Did you ever shave?' I must have been one of the highlights of my gynaecologist's career.

45–46: gynaecologist retired, after prescribing new tablets – Premarin – a more natural way of taking oestrogen. She referred me to my GP for future care.

I did not like Premarin. I felt my complexion was 'yellow' and I developed occasional blemishes and dry patches on my face, which I had never had before. I lost weight and could not regain it. Now my GP was seeing me, my blood pressure was checked and found to be extremely high (205/95). Several treatments were tried and after three years it came down to 170/80.

49: my husband and I watched a BBC programme, *Dark Secret*, about XY women with androgen insensitivity syndrome and everything fell into place. I was not alone . . . I contacted the AIS Support Group and tried to contact my gynaecologist only to find she had recently died. I had a new GP and wrote, requesting a long session to go through my medical records, which we did. It was a harrowing though liberating experience to finally put the jigsaw pieces together. It would have been a great help to have known the facts many years earlier. (Throughout my adult life my condition has made me feel isolated and I have avoided close friendships with either sex, especially when my contemporaries were busy having families.)

Through the AIS Support Group, I became aware of HRT patches and started on Estraderm. Immediately my skin improved and I gained weight (now I need to lose some!). My blood pressure has fallen and I feel so much better than before. Some of this may also be due to a new inner calm as a result of meeting others with the same condition. I've also had a bone scan (never previously suggested) and my X-rays proved more than satisfactory.

One of the techniques I have employed to face the reality of AIS is to create my own 'workshop manual' with sections containing: the version of events I was told; family snapshots of myself during my life together with personal recollections of experiences relating to my condition; and information on what I now know actually happened – gleaned from my medical files and other literature. It also has all the AIS Support Group newsletters.

What of the future? I have recently told some long-term friends about my condition and they were very understanding. I want to maintain contact with the AIS Support Group for my own sense of 'belonging' and to help other women (and possibly the medical profession too). I believe society needs to be awakened to the existence and acceptance of intersex conditions and, who knows, I might even write my own book!

2

BODY CHEMISTRY

The menopause occurs when the ovaries run out of follicles. Usually this happens mid-life, but it can occur earlier. This chapter takes a look at women's bodies to see where follicles come into the picture and how the eggs and sex hormones they produce fit into the menstrual cycle. It also explains how these hormones work and why drugs and substances that mimic hormones can alter women's body chemistry.

A New Look

The diagram below (2.1) is probably nothing new. What may come as a surprise is that it is the uterus viewed from behind, not from the front!

That may seem a little odd. It is hardly the angle to help women visualize themselves! However, doctors illustrate the uterus from the rear to show the Fallopian tubes and ovaries, which tend to straggle up *behind* it in reality. This arrangement is much easier to understand from the side view in Figure 2.2.

Other aspects of these diagrams are worth a second look. For example, referring to Figure 2.1, one could be forgiven for thinking that the vagina was like a short length of hose-pipe. Instead, its elastic walls lie closed like a soft glove. At rest, it has an average length of 10 cm, which elongates during sexual arousal. Very occasionally, however, women are born with short vaginas.

Figure 2.1 also suggests that the vagina goes straight up to where the uterus sits above it, like a head on a neck. However, the vagina slopes

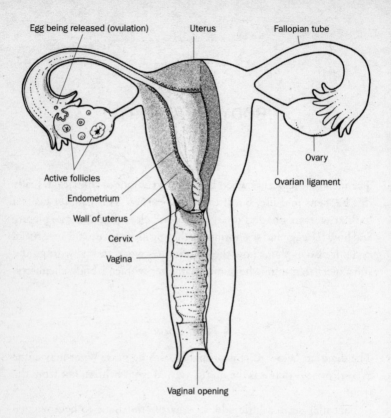

Figure 2.1 Looking from behind

backwards into the body until it meets the uterus, which slopes forward at a right angle. This angle means the uterus opens into the *side* of the top of the vagina. This is easier to see in Figure 2.2. Yet, even here, all is not as it seems: 20 per cent of women have a 'retroverted' uterus which rests back against the bowel rather than forward over the bladder. Usually this is just the way the uterus happens to lie, although retroversion can be caused by scar tissue (adhesions) due to pelvic inflammatory disease, endometriosis or surgery.

After puberty the uterus becomes the size and shape of an upside-

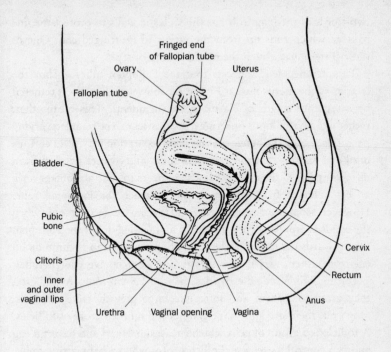

Ovary

Fringed end
of Fallopian tube

Uterus

Fallopian tube

Bladder

Pubic
bone

Clitoris

Inner
and outer
vaginal lips

Urethra

Vaginal opening

Vagina

Cervix

Rectum

Anus

Figure 2.2 Looking from the side

down pear (Figure 2.1). Its muscular walls are about 2 cm thick and lined by a special layer (the endometrium), which grows and is shed during the menstrual cycle. The walls touch each other leaving a triangular hollow about the width of a fingernail. This tiny hollow may seem surprising since many diagrams suggest a larger cavity. Sometimes women have a divided or double uterus and/or vagina.

The hollow of the uterus has three openings: one down through the cervix into the vagina and two up into the Fallopian tubes. The cervix is a small cone at the top of the vagina. The cervix is often described as feeling like the rubbery tip of the nose or chin; the latter if one has had children. The Fallopian tubes rise up and back behind the uterus. Each tube is about the width of a pencil and about two-thirds of the length. It has thick elastic walls to protect the fine passage which runs up from the uterus to its fringed end. One of these fringes may clutch the neighbouring ovary.

This arrangement suggests that the Fallopian tubes anchor the ovaries to the uterus but, as Figure 2.1 shows, each ovary is tethered by a separate length of elastic tissue (ligament). This means that, rather like two balloons on strings, the ovaries can be found in varying positions among the pelvic organs. This separation may seem curious until one realizes that the Fallopian tubes and ovaries develop from different parts of the embryo. It also appears to pose a problem since an egg released from the ovary has to reach the Fallopian tube. However, separation is temporary and the gap can be overcome when the egg is catapulted from the ovary and ferried down the Fallopian tube towards the uterus. Indeed, a Fallopian tube can vacuum up an egg from either ovary if necessary (e.g. if women have a single tube).

During childhood, the ovaries may be 1.5 cm long. At puberty, they grow to 3.5 cm and look like large greyish-white almonds. However, their size and shape can depend on their store of follicles. A follicle is a group of cells which encases, protects and feeds an egg and can control its release. Follicles form when a baby girl is in her mother's womb. By the fifth month of pregnancy, a baby's ovaries have created all the eggs she may need for *her* children. By the time she is born, her body has cleared out two-thirds of this supply (for unknown reasons) and enclosed many of the remaining eggs within individual follicles.

Once in place, the supply of egg follicles cannot be renewed in any way. So, if egg follicles do not develop before birth, a woman may have no ovaries or 'streak' ovaries. If the store of follicles is low, she may have small ovaries and/or a premature menopause.

The Menstrual Cycle

The basic pattern of each menstrual cycle is fairly simple. The ovarian follicles are stimulated until one of them releases an egg which travels down the nearby Fallopian tube to the uterus. During this time the lining of the uterus thickens to receive and feed the egg, if it becomes fertilized by a sperm. If pregnancy does not occur, the egg passes out of the body and the lining is shed at a period about 14 days later.

The body chemistry which controls the menstrual cycle is rather more complicated (and not yet fully understood). However, order and timing are everything. For example, the lining of the uterus must be ready by the time the egg is released. Otherwise, if the egg becomes fertilized, it won't settle and grow. Similarly the lining must not be shed too early, otherwise any pregnancy will be lost.

Four parts of the body interact to ensure that things go according to plan. Two have already been mentioned: an active ovarian follicle and the lining of the uterus. The other two are a bean-sized area of the brain, called the hypothalamus, and its pea-sized neighbour, the pituitary gland. Each part does something different, but together they act towards the same goal: making pregnancy possible, month after month.

The hypothalamus is often described as the conductor of the menstrual orchestra or like the thermostat in a central heating system. These analogies suggest that it is in charge and therefore less influenced by other parts. However, this is somewhat misleading because the ovarian follicles are just as influential once the menstrual cycle is in full swing. For example, unlike a radiator and thermostat, an active follicle can alter the *setting* of the hypothalamus. Perhaps it is more helpful to think of the hypothalamus, pituitary gland, uterus and ovarian follicles as equal members of a team that adjust constantly to the overall state of play.[1] They do this by releasing and responding to each other's hormones.

Hormonal interactions begin in late childhood. A pulse generator in the hypothalamus times spurts of gonadotrophin-releasing hormone (GnRH) into the bloodstream. At first, pulses of hormone occur every so often at night, but then they start to appear during the day too. Slowly GnRH stimulates the nearby pituitary gland to release spurts of follicle-stimulating hormone (FSH), which are carried to the distant ovaries. As its name suggests, FSH is designed to stimulate follicles.

As FSH blood levels rise, some of the waiting egg follicles respond with low levels of oestradiol (main type of oestrogen). Oestradiol enlarges the womb and thickens its lining. It also affects the vagina so that it can become wet during sexual excitement. In fact, oestradiol is responsible for many of the changes at puberty. However, it is also the ovaries' signal to the hypothalamus and pituitary gland that egg follicles have been stimulated. In response, FSH production slows down.

Active follicles do not last long. As they die off, oestradiol levels fall and the signal changes. More FSH is produced to stimulate another group of follicles and so on. Eventually the lining of the uterus has thickened enough for a girl to have her first period when her oestradiol levels fall during the next hormonal fluctuation. However, the hormonal swings are not strong enough for her follicles to release an egg yet.

It can take many cycles before the hypothalamus's pulse generator reaches an adult setting (spurts every 90 minutes).[2] When it does, it prompts the pituitary to release a mature level of FSH. This stimulates the most active egg follicle to produce more oestradiol, which sets the stage for ovulation. The new peak in oestradiol jacks up the setting on the pulse generator. The extra spurts of GnRH tell the pituitary gland to release a new substance into the bloodstream: luteinizing hormone (LH). The surge in LH makes the active follicle burst to release its egg (ovulation).

Looking at the run-up to ovulation, one can see that a group of follicles produces oestradiol to thicken the lining of the uterus in preparation for an egg. When this hormone reaches a peak, signalling that the most active follicle is ready, there is a surge of LH – the very hormone needed to make that follicle ovulate. It is almost as if the ripest apple shakes the tree when it is ready to fall!

It is often thought that the ovaries take it in turns to ovulate, but it seems to be a simple race among the follicles activated that month. The fittest follicle wins, whichever ovary it happens to be in. Having

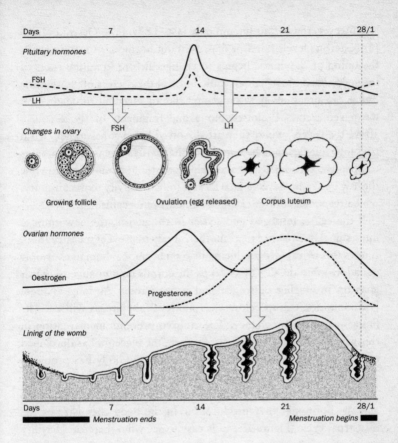

Figure 2.3 The menstrual cycle

released its egg, the follicle sac becomes bright yellow and is called the corpus luteum ('body yellow'). The corpus luteum still provides oestradiol, although less than before. However, it isn't just a different colour; it has a different job. Stimulated by LH, it also produces the hormone progesterone. Progesterone signals to the uterus that an egg has been released. The uterus responds by filling the lining with secretions which can nourish an egg, if it is fertilized.

However, the corpus luteum only lasts a few days. Oestradiol and progesterone levels fall as it dies. Without hormones to stimulate it, the lining of the uterus begins to change. Before long, the roots of the specialized blood vessels kink and seal themselves off so that the lining can break away without any risk of bleeding to death – no mean achievement! Clotted blood and fragments of tissue collect above the cervix, where they are dissolved by enzymes to help them pass into the vagina. The muscles of the uterus increase contractions to open the cervix slightly and help expel the remnants. Meanwhile the low oestradiol levels signal lack of follicle activity to the pituitary, which responds with FSH and so a new cycle begins.

If the egg *is* fertilized and settles in the uterus, the new embryo must signal its presence to its mother's body to prevent menstruation. It does this by rapidly producing its own hormone: human chorionic gonadotrophin (hCG). hCG keeps the corpus luteum alive so that it goes on producing oestrogen and progesterone. As long as these hormones don't drop below a certain level, the uterus will keep its lining – and the pregnancy. The embryo prevents menstruation in this way for about seven weeks. By then, the placenta has developed enough to take over this job. Occasionally, the body has problems juggling this changeover and miscarriage occurs.

The menopause occurs when the ovaries run out of egg follicles and the hormones they produce. Given the body chemistry of the menstrual cycle (Figure 2.3), it is easy to see why, therefore, fertility and periods would come to an end.

How Hormones Work

Often women have heard of oestrogen and progesterone, the hormones produced by an active egg follicle. Usually they have also heard of testosterone. However, what one tends to hear is that oestrogen and progesterone are the female sex hormones and testosterone is the male sex hormone. This is somewhat misleading because men can produce oestrogen and women can produce testosterone. It is more

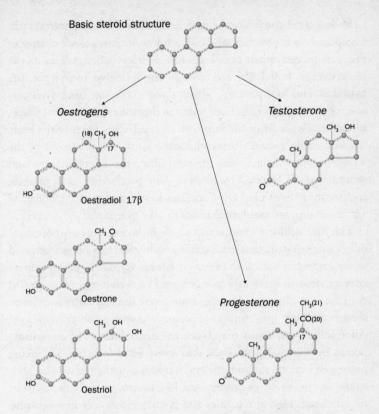

Basic steroid structure

Oestrogens

Testosterone

(18) CH₃ OH
17

HO

Oestradiol 17β

Oestrone

HO

CH₃ O

HO

CH₃ OH OH

HO

Oestriol

Progesterone CH₃(21)
CH₃ CO(20)
17

CH₃

O

Figure 2.4 Sex hormones have a similar chemical structure

accurate to see oestrogens as the feminizing hormones. Testosterone is one of the masculinizing hormones (androgens).

As Figure 2.4 shows, the sex hormones have the same chemical framework: four rings of hydrocarbon molecules (represented by geometric shapes). The slightly different letters labelling the edges of these rings are chemical codes for side groups of carbon, hydrogen and oxygen atoms attached to the four rings. The details do not really matter here. What is of more interest is the fact that these different side groups give each sex hormone a distinctive molecular *shape*.

Molecular shape is like the pattern of a key. By fitting into certain 'receptors' on the surface of a cell, a hormone can unlock change in that cell. Indeed, when an ovarian follicle releases oestradiol into the bloodstream, it unlocks receptors in the lining of the uterus, the hypothalamus and pituitary gland – and that's just for starters, as oestrogen receptors have been found in the heart, bone, breast tissue, blood vessels, areas of the brain, etc. Yet different parts of the body respond in their own way to the same hormone: the lining of the womb thickens in response to oestradiol, the hypothalamus and pituitary gland respond by altering their production of hormones, and so on. In each case, the 'lock-and-key' fit between the hormone and the receptors enables reactions to take place.

The 'lock-and-key' mechanism also helps to explain how hormonal drugs work. A drug that has a structure identical to a hormone found in the body can unlock change as if it were a spare key. Drugs with enough structural resemblance can act like skeleton keys and 'pick' the receptor, causing change as if they were the real hormone – even though the body may not have encountered such a substance before. Alternatively impostors may block the usual changes by preventing access by the real key. They may even act *selectively*, unlocking oestrogen receptors in some organs but blocking them elsewhere. For example, 'designer' oestrogens act like oestrogen in bone, but not breast tissue. Herbal remedies and certain substances in foods also appear to act as skeleton keys.

The idea of structural similarity and 'hormone-like' effects is cropping up in descriptions for all sorts of products. However, structural similarity is not a guarantee that a substance will work in the body or act as hoped. A roughly similar compound can unlock or 'pick' a receptor, but a slight difference can be enough to spoil the fit. The difference may be nothing more than a side chain that sticks out at an unsuitable angle or a mirror image structure that matches like a glove on the wrong hand.

The body makes use of the fact that a small structural change can produce a different effect when it converts one sex hormone into another (Figure 2.5). Indeed, they are all made from the same starting

Figure 2.5 How the body makes sex hormones (simplified)

Cholesterol

▼

Progesterone

▼

Androstenedione (adrenal hormone)

▼

Testosterone

▼

Oestradiol

block, cholesterol. One can almost imagine this as a TV demonstration of a recipe. First take cholesterol, add a few enzymes to change the side chains to progesterone, followed by a quick enzyme snip here to get androstenedione, and again for testosterone before the final stir and out of the pot comes the rearranged form: oestradiol. Cells stop at the relevant stages of the recipe depending on the substance which they are due to release. For example, cells in the corpus luteum complete the steps to progesterone; cells in the adrenal glands go as far as androstenedione; the egg follicles go all the way through to oestradiol.

The TV demonstration has a serious side since drug companies have used Nature's recipes to make sex hormones or related drugs. For example, scientists discovered that plant substances in yams and soy beans with a similar molecular structure (Figures 2.4 and 4.2 on p. 62) can be converted into progesterone in the laboratory (the body *cannot* convert plants into natural progesterone, Chapter 11). From there, other sex hormones can be produced by altering the side groups. Furthermore, by creating side groups with molecular arrangements not found in Nature, drug companies can produce synthetic sex hormones that can be patented for profit. For instance, the contraceptive pill contains a synthetic form of oestrogen (ethinyl oestradiol) that has a much stronger effect than natural oestrogens and can change the chemistry of the menstrual cycle to prevent pregnancy. Hormone replacement therapy may contain natural or synthetic hormones which also act on the body's chemistry.

3

NATURAL MENOPAUSE

'As long as I knew what was happening to my body I was satisfied and did not worry. I found that whenever I started to feel hot, but relaxed, I "cooled down" immediately.'

WALTRAUD

What happens when the menopausal body-clock is triggered and the ovaries run out of egg follicles? This chapter describes the hormonal changes that lead to the natural menopause and the symptoms that they may – or may not – cause. Many apparent symptoms are still a matter of debate. Indeed, the final period is the only recognizable sign of change that women share in the natural menopause! Women's experiences vary enormously, as shown by the stories here and in Chapter 1.

Menopausal Body-clock

Like mother, like daughter. It is often said that a woman will have her menopause at much the same age as her mother did. Or that women who begin their periods early will finish late. However, researchers haven't found much truth in these sayings.[1] What they have found is that the average age for the menopause has not changed much down the centuries and is remarkably similar in different parts of the world. In contrast, the age at which girls begin their periods has fallen in industrialized countries, probably due to improved health.

Scientists think that women approach the menopause when their supply of egg follicles falls below about 1000. Women cannot produce eggs every day, like men produce sperm. Instead they are born with a store of 400–500,000 follicles.[2] This appears to be more than enough: only 0.01 per cent are ever ovulated.[3] However, numerous additional follicles become active each cycle and then fade away. Yet more disappear steadily over the years. But even this loss doesn't add up. Now researchers have realized that the supply falls to 1000 because most of the follicles suddenly die off in a change triggered by some kind of menopausal body-clock.

No one really knows why this 'follicle clearance' occurs or whether anything can be done to prevent it. Although the menopause seems unnecessary, some biologists think that it evolved to protect women and their existing offspring from the risks of further pregnancies. Whatever the reason, the menopausal body-clock means that most women are reduced to a similarly low number of follicles and begin the hormonal changes which result in their last period at much the same time of life.

Usually women stop menstruating between the ages of 48 and 55. In the UK the average age is 51. However, the menopause can be up to two years earlier for women who smoke. Doctors have also realized that the menopause is brought forward by up to four years in 25 per cent of women who have a hysterectomy and keep at least one ovary during surgery (see page 175). The menopause is defined as premature if it is before the age of 40, but this age limit is a handy round number rather than anything more significant. Some doctors feel that this definition should be extended because women who experience the menopause before the age of 45 have an extra risk of heart disease and osteoporosis.[4]

A premature menopause can occur at almost any age. Often the reasons are unknown. It may be due to a short supply of egg follicles or because the menopausal body-clock was triggered too soon. It may be because a woman's ovaries have been removed or damaged during surgery or cancer treatment. If this loss takes place after puberty, it will cause the menopause. If it takes place before, women will need hormone replacement therapy to go through puberty and begin menstruation, if possible. This treatment will not restore fertility.

Hormonal Count-down

Hormonal changes begin sometime after the body-clock has triggered the sudden 'stock clearance' of egg follicles. The remaining follicles appear to be increasingly unresponsive to stimulation. The pituitary gland tries to remedy this by releasing extra FSH each month. Overall, levels of FSH start to rise like a tide, even though individual waves of FSH still fluctuate from day to day and cycle to cycle.

The first thing women may notice is more frequent periods, perhaps every 21 days or so.[5] This can happen in their mid-forties or earlier. Cycle length drops because the first half of the cycle (when FSH is released) shortens. This shift can come as a surprise or worry. Women may expect less frequent periods, if anything! But some women will find that their periods get closer together before becoming further apart. Others won't experience any change at this stage.

As time goes on, the dwindling supply of responsive egg follicles means that women become less fertile. Well over a third of women aged 45–50 have cycles which skip ovulation.[6] If an egg is not released, there will be no corpus luteum (follicle sac left behind) to produce progesterone that month. This can lead to a heavier period because the lining of the womb continues to thicken in response to oestradiol, but without the balancing effects of progesterone during the last half of the cycle.

Women can also have an unexpectedly heavy flow if the lining builds up because a period is delayed. In this case, irregular heavy bleeding is part of menopausal changes, but women should check with their doctor if it continues because it can also be a sign of uterine problems, e.g. endometrial hyperplasia (unwanted growth of the womb lining associated with endometrical cancer), fibroids, etc.[7] Again, experience differs: numerous women find that their blood loss remains unchanged at this stage or becomes scanty.

On average, women have irregular periods for about four years before they come to an end. One in 10 women stop suddenly (see Eileen, Chapter 1).[8] For others, menstruation can be erratic for five years or more before stopping altogether. One study found that less than half of the women aged 45–49 years who lacked periods for six months had actually had the menopause.[9] Of those who stopped for 12 months, 10 per cent menstruated again.

In the years before the final period, the tide of FSH rises as the pituitary tries to kick-start the remaining follicles, whereas the tide of progesterone falls as ovulation becomes less frequent. The other hormones fluctuate much as before. Then, as follicles become scarce, the pituitary hormone LH increases three- to fivefold and oestradiol levels fall. Without adequate stimulation by oestradiol, the lining of the womb does not grow and is no longer shed.

Oestradiol levels drop by up to 80 per cent in the year or so after periods end. However, hormonal fluctuations can continue for some time and the last few follicles may yet respond. For this reason, doctors advise women over 50 to use contraception for 12 months after their periods finish. Women under 50 are advised to use contraception for two years after an apparent menopause.

In these days of hi-tech medicine, it can seem surprising that there is no quick, simple, reliable test to predict when women will have their last period – or whether they have had it – or when those flushes will stop! However, hormone levels vary enormously for the same woman at different times and even at the same time during different cycles. So doctors tend to judge whether a woman is in the menopause by her symptoms and the pattern of her periods. The general rule is that a woman who has not had periods for 12 months is post-menopausal.

This guideline isn't much help for women who have had a hysterectomy. If in doubt, GPs can check blood FSH levels which rise in response to lack of responsive egg follicles. This is better than measuring oestradiol levels, which fall at such a late stage (Figure 3.1). However, as explained in Chapter 7, FSH levels are not a foolproof test because the ovaries can revive temporarily and post-menopausal FSH readings have been found in women who were still having regular periods![10]

Figure 3.1 Hormonal count-down

The changes during the menopause are the result of a complex biological process winding down over time. In many ways, it is the reverse of what took place during puberty when the hormonal themes were elaborated upon until everything was in full swing.

- Changes begin when the number of egg follicles falls below about 1,000. The remaining follicles appear to be less responsive.
- The pituitary gland produces more FSH (follicle-stimulating hormone), perhaps to try and kick-start the remaining follicles.
- Extra FSH can lead to shorter cycles. Women may notice this in their early forties, although many women experience no particular change at this stage.
- Lack of responsive follicles can lead to lack of ovulation during a cycle.
- No ovulation means no progesterone is produced that month. This is one reason why a period can be heavier than expected.
- Delayed menstruation is also likely to be heavier as the lining builds up during the delay.
- Alternatively, periods can become scanty and irregular. They can be a fortnight or several months apart.
- As the supply of responsive follicles comes to an end, women produce less oestradiol. At the time of the last period and for about a year afterwards, oestradiol levels drop by about 80 per cent.[11]
- Symptoms such as hot flushes appear at this stage for many women, although they may begin earlier when women miss the odd period.
- Women are regarded as post-menopausal if they have not menstruated for at least 12 months.
- The slowly rising tide of FSH reaches its height two to three years after the last period. At this stage, it is 10–15 times greater than when change began. The tide falls over the next 20–30 years.
- The ovaries still release some oestradiol. Oestrone, a weaker type of oestrogen, is also produced elsewhere, particularly adipose tissue (a type of body fat).
- The ovaries produce 20 per cent less testosterone.

Menopausal Symptoms

Joint aches and pains, anxiety and depression, irritability, insomnia, forgetfulness, feeling weepy, bad headaches and breast tenderness. One in 10 women aged 47 reported that they were 'bothered a lot' by these problems in a recent survey.[12] Less commonly reported at this age were troublesome hot flushes (7 per cent), night sweats (6 per cent) and vaginal dryness (4.2 per cent), although these are likely to increase as more women become post-menopausal in this group. Other occasional mentions included pins and needles, skin crawling and hair loss.

Hot flushes, night sweats and vaginal dryness are the only symptoms on this list that can be related directly to the hormonal changes described in the previous section. Beyond this, one gets into a lot of debate. When is a menopausal symptom a menopausal symptom and when is it a reaction to changing experience, life events or simply a sign of ageing?

The answer can depend on how one chooses to understand the menopause. For example, many doctors see menopausal symptoms as being due to lack of oestrogen, which can be remedied by HRT. Others argue that the menopause is not a deficiency disease and many so-called symptoms are due to other aspects of women's lives at the time, rather than the state of their hormones. If one takes this view, then medical treatment with HRT cannot be the solution.

This may seem confusing; surely the evidence points one way or the other? However, although much is understood about ovarian follicles and hormonal changes during the menopause, less is known about the physical effects of these changes. After all, there is only one universal symptom that women share: their periods end. Other apparent symptoms vary enormously for different women and across different cultures, suggesting that lifestyle and the social and personal meanings of the menopause can influence women's physical experiences of this change. In addition, the effects of HRT on many of these symptoms are difficult to unravel and are still largely debatable.

Of course, all this supposes that 'symptoms' are a problem.

Undoubtedly they are for women attending clinics, who are frequently studied by researchers. However, several large surveys in the UK, USA and Canada have followed representative groups of women through the menopause. They found that although many women experienced 'symptoms' as their periods came to an end and for some time thereafter, few women had great difficulties. Indeed, some researchers have questioned the negative stereotypes of the menopause that abound because they give women unnecessarily worrying expectations.[13] One GP has commented that women often attend the surgery with what they perceive to be menopausal problems but prove to be something else.[14] Equally, stereotypes may lead doctors to prescribe HRT unnecessarily and women to have unrealistic expectations of treatment.[15]

Hot flushes and night sweats

Hot flushes and night sweats can begin when a woman starts to miss the odd period; they may even be mistaken for premenstrual tension.[16] However, they are far more likely just before periods stop altogether and thereafter. Estimates of how many women get hot flushes vary. In Western countries, perhaps 65 per cent of women have hot flushes, although most women are not too troubled by them. For example, only 20 per cent request help from their doctor in Britain. A large American project found that women were more likely to be bothered about irregular bleeding.[17] Meanwhile, as is often quoted these days, Japanese women appear to be comparatively free of hot flushes and the concept does not exist as such in the Japanese language.

This may be depressing reading for women who feel plagued. Certainly some women suffer 50 or more flushes a day, several an hour. Frequent or severe flushing can be very difficult to manage in public situations and night sweats may be an added misery, regularly disrupting sleep. In some cases, women suffer for several months until the temporary return of periods brings a spell of relief (see Audrey, Chapter 1). Most women find that their symptoms ease 1–2 years after periods finish, although 25 per cent of women have them for longer. Occasionally, women still get flushes more than five years later.[18]

Hot flushes and night sweats are called vasomotor symptoms because they occur when blood vessels (vaso-) dilate or constrict (-motor). Hot flushes can vary from mild, not unpleasant, feelings of warmth to what Audrey called the 'hot clammy' kind. Severe hot flushes often begin as sudden heat in the neck which spreads up over the face and scalp and down across the chest. Many women say they can recognize when one is about to start because they get a funny feeling moments before. This may be due to the rapid increase in heartbeat and flow of blood to the skin as the body attempts to cool itself. Women can become red-faced and show visible signs of sweat, although usually this feels a lot worse than it looks. Some women also get palpitations or may feel dizzy. Typically a flush lasts about three minutes, although it can feel like a lot longer! Occasionally it *is* a lot longer: a flush can continue for up to an hour.

Scientists have tried to understand what happens during a hot flush by measuring levels of various substances, blood pressure, skin temperature, sweating and even 'core' temperature, which is recorded by asking women to swallow a radiotelemetry capsule. The results show that women's core temperature usually rises slightly before a hot flush (although it can fall).[19] During the flush, blood flow at the fingertips may be 4–30 times greater[20] and skin temperature can be an extra 1–5°C.[21] That said, it seems that women only experience the initial rise in temperature as 'the flush' because the feeling disappears within minutes, compared to the 20–40 minutes it takes the body to return to normal. Women can also feel themselves to be much hotter than indicated by temperature readings.

The experience of women who have had their ovaries removed suggests that hot flushes are something to do with oestrogen. Their symptoms can be severe, but are treatable with HRT. However, low oestrogen levels cannot be the simple reason because women who experience hot flushes in the natural menopause can have *higher* oestrogen levels than women who do not. Now researchers think that falling oestrogen is what matters rather than the actual level. A fall may disturb the hypothalamus in the brain, which in turn upsets the nearby thermoregulatory centre. When triggered, this centre prompts the changes described above as if there was a need to cool the body. Hormone therapy may treat hot flushes and night sweats by providing fairly even levels of oestrogen (although see implants, Chapter 10).

The thermoregulatory centre only seems to behave this way if sensitized by enough oestrogen in the first place (usually at puberty).[22] Sensitization would explain why teenagers who lack ovarian hormones due to a genetic problem or a premature menopause can be free of hot flushes before taking HRT and yet be surprised by symptoms if they stop treatment at a later stage (see Susan, Chapter 7). Coming off HRT suddenly causes falling oestrogen levels that are thought to trigger hot flushes in sensitized women. Therefore doctors advise women to taper their HRT to reduce possible withdrawal symptoms.

Vaginal dryness, urinary problems and waning libido

Vaginal dryness can occur for different reasons and 26 per cent of women report this problem *before* the menopause.[23] However, there is reasonable agreement that vaginal dryness is more likely after the menopause because women have less oestrogen. This may result in reduced blood flow and lubrication, which can reduce women's sexual confidence in turn (see Maureen, below). Vaginal tissue can be more vulnerable to lack of lubrication as it becomes thinner and less elastic. Occasionally severe symptoms can develop such as burning, itching, pain or bleeding. The urethra also becomes more vulnerable and women may find that sex triggers the need to go to the toilet more often or bouts of cystitis.

After the menopause, the vagina loses some of its acidity and resistance to bacteria. This may explain why some women are more prone to urinary infections at this stage. The problem appears to be hormone-related and can be reversed by vaginal oestrogen cream, but it can also improve with vaginal gels which aim to restore the acidity rather than the hormones. In contrast, the need to go to the toilet more often or being unable to get there in time does not benefit from hormone treatment. Pelvic floor exercises are advised for women with urinary incontinence (see page 275).

The effect of the menopause on libido is far more difficult to assess and, perhaps not surprisingly, studies have led to conflicting results. The menopause could have positive effects by relieving women of periods and, after a time, the need for contraception (see page 34). It could also have negative effects as a result of vaginal dryness or, more indirectly, because of other symptoms. For example, night sweats and insomnia may lead to tiredness and irritability, which are unlikely to improve one's sex life. Obviously libido can depend on a lot of things; not least, whether one has a partner, how one feels in the relationship and any problems *they* may or may not have. Indeed, the most significant effect on women's sex lives after the menopause is the way they were before.[24] Most women's experiences are not altered significantly and any problems during the menopause are likely to be temporary.[25] Later women may be affected by the loss of a partner, ageing and ill-health, but these effects need to be separated from the menopause as such.

However, some researchers think that loss of libido may be explained by testosterone deficiency. This view is based on observations that women who have their ovaries removed often complain of sexual difficulties, which do not improve until testosterone is added to their oestrogen therapy. It is not clear to what extent these findings apply to women who have had a natural menopause. After such surgery, testosterone levels fall by 50 per cent. The fall is much less after the natural menopause. Although testosterone is no longer released by egg follicles, it is still made by other ovarian cells and elsewhere. However, some researchers have argued that there is an age-related decline in testosterone levels which may have a significant effect on libido in time.

Forgetfulness

It is often said that women become forgetful during the menopause, although few studies have investigated whether this is so. Memory lapses may be nothing more than a knock-on effect of coping with insomnia and stress due to symptoms such as flushes and sweats. However, a few researchers have been interested in the possibility of a hormonal link.[26] They gave women who had had their ovaries removed memory tests in the first two months after surgery. Half the women received oestrogen therapy, half received a placebo. The study also took into account other symptoms that might disrupt the results. Both groups performed visual and attention tests without difficulties, but in time the women on placebo did less well on the verbal memory tests. It is not clear how these results apply to women in the natural menopause who experience a gradual 80 per cent fall in oestradiol rather than a sudden complete loss.

Forgetfulness during the menopause can be frightening (see Jan, below), given the publicity that oestrogen therapy may help prevent Alzheimer's disease. This is an understandable concern, but the study that attracted media attention was done in women in their seventies.[27] Older women may wonder if they should consider HRT for this reason, but few doctors would recommend HRT to them on the grounds of this study alone. Research is still at an early stage.

Mood swings and depression

The idea that the menopause is associated with depression is not new. It can be traced back to the Victorian belief that women's psychiatric state is linked to their reproductive system. Such ideas die hard; first described in 1906, involutional melancholia was only removed from official disease classifications as recently as 1980.[28]

In the meantime all sorts of studies have shown all sorts of associations between all sorts of psychological symptoms and the menopause. In many cases questions arise as to how this research was done and whether the participants were representative of women in general.

In the end, as several reviewers have pointed out, there is little evidence that the menopause is related to any psychological symptoms compared to the link found between the menopause and hot flushes.

Studies that have followed groups of women in the community through their experiences have found few associations between the menopause and depression.[29] Women who were depressed at this time were more likely to be women who had suffered depression before, had fears about the menopause or were coping with stressful life events. Other research suggests that women who have a lengthy menopause can become depressed for a while – perhaps understandably!

These findings suggest that psychological symptoms during the menopause are not hormone-related. However, HRT is described as providing a mental tonic. This may be partly a direct effect of oestrogen, but it may also be that HRT promotes well-being by alleviating undermining symptoms such as night sweats and insomnia.[30]

Headaches

A few women get what are known as menstrual migraines: severe headaches triggered a day or two before a period but at no other time. This is different from other types of migraine that occur earlier in the cycle and improve at this stage! Researchers have found that menstrual migraines are associated with falling oestrogen, which may explain why they are more common in women aged 35–45, who are experiencing hormonal changes in the run-up to the menopause.[31] Often this type of migraine eases after the menopause, if hormones were the cause. A research trial of 360 mg/day magnesium suggests that supplements may help prevent attacks. If not, menstrual migraines can improve on HRT, although other women get bad headaches for the first time on hormone treatment.[32]

Women's Stories

Waltraud

I was born on August 2, 1928. I was a late starter with menstruation at the age of 14, which in those days was actually thought to be quite normal (my mother was 16 when her first period began and she finished in her mid-fifties without any problems).

My periods stopped when I was about 53, but started again six months later and continued for another year. Some time after they had stopped altogether, I got my first hot flushes. I consulted my doctor to find out why this had occurred and was told that the production of hormones was decreasing, but this was not gradual. She said that this would happen every so often and reduce in bouts.

As long as I knew what was happening to my body I was satisfied and did not worry. I found that whenever I started to feel hot, but relaxed, I 'cooled down' immediately. From my German medical books I knew that certain herbs could be helpful in the menopause, particularly teas made from dried wild strawberry leaves. In German chemists and herbal shops you can buy this for the purpose.

I had a very easy time. Relaxation, an optimistic outlook on life, a very happy marriage and my four wonderful children must all have helped me to lead a happy life.

Jan (Australia)

I was 48 years old when the bloody menopause (pun intended!) turned my life upside-down!

I had never had period problems, had sailed through one miscarriage and two pregnancies and was secretly quite proud of my ability to cope well with being a woman and all that it entailed.

The Pill had not suited me when I tried it as a 20-year-old – I got too moody and had very sore swollen breasts – so I used a diaphragm cap in the early years of marriage and then had an IUD until I had my tubes tied. I was very confident that when I did go through the menopause it would be a breeze and I would probably not even realize it was happening. How wrong I was.

It began with my periods becoming irregular both in their spacing and the time they lasted. I would find myself hot all over (not a flush) when other people were not. I began having headaches regularly – something that had been rare for me previously. I became moody – sometimes so depressed I would feel suicidal – and that brought feelings of guilt because I was having a great life (better than in previous years) and had nothing to be depressed about! The fact that my children had grown up and were mostly off my hands was wonderful as far as I was concerned and I couldn't understand the empty-nest syndrome. I was getting involved in things that interested me and really enjoying the freedom to do that.

By far the worst symptom for me was the short-term memory loss – I was truly afraid I was heading for Alzheimer's disease. Because my hair started to fall out too, I had tests for thyroid problems and my thyroid was found to be overactive. Eventually I had radium treatment for this. I had a bone-density check and that was OK.

My doctor put me on HRT: Premarin 0.625 mg and Provera 0.5 mg. I complained about sore breasts for 7–10 days before my period and depression and nine months later was changed to Triquilar ED. My breasts were even more tender on that, so I went back to Premarin.

I struggled on but was still not OK, so I went off HRT for several months. The old menopausal symptoms returned gradually and a year later I decided to try a different type of HRT. Within months my periods were all over the place, so I changed to Trisequens, Navidrex (for water retention) and evening primrose oil (for breast tenderness). The first few months were OK, then the sore breasts recurred and became unbearable so I gave up HRT again.

By the following year the symptoms were back and the memory loss was frightening me, so I tried Trisequens again. Within months the sore breasts were unbearable and my periods irregular, so I reverted to Premarin/Provera. The Premarin dose was reduced to 0.3 mg and I started Oroxin for my thyroid, which had become underactive after the radium treatment.

That New Year, I can remember feeling desperate – my breasts were so sore I would cradle them in my hands when I turned over in bed at night – it was like shifting hot bricks on my chest! I asked for referral to a specialist – an endocrinologist.

She explained that we would have to experiment, that all women are different in their HRT requirements and that because sore breasts had been a pattern for me for most of my life it would not be easy and perhaps not possible to completely eradicate that side-effect.

She prescribed an eight-week course of evening primrose oil 3000 mg (3 g) a day with Vitamin B1 and B6 but no HRT in that time. Then I began a lower dose of Premarin and on days 12–26, a lower dose of Primolut N.*

There was still some breast soreness after a few months so I eventually settled on taking Premarin on alternate days. The headaches were one symptom that continued and got worse, so that by the following year they had become like a migraine and I would end up vomiting. There was some connection with a neck problem, but it also seemed connected with my cycle, so my doctor suggested that I take Primolut N continually (see page 222) alongside the Premarin – thereby eliminating my periods. Wonderful!

That was last year and I have continued that regime with no breast soreness. In effect, it took five and a half years to sort out the best treatment for me. I am happy (and relieved!) to say that I now feel well and *normal* and I have also found other ways to cope with the headaches – lots of smiles, yoga exercises and the occasional aspirin.

* Dose lowering should be done by a doctor as women need enough progestogen in combined HRT to oppose the oestrogen and protect against the extra risk of endometrial cancer. Also, while some lower doses may be enough to prevent menopausal symptoms, a certain minimum is required if women want to prevent osteoporosis as well (see Figure 10.1, page 214).

Maureen

I am 57 and the main problem for me has been vaginal dryness. The menopause wasn't anything out of the ordinary. My periods got irregular and I had some hot flushes, but nothing that troubled me much. That was several years ago now and, to be honest, I hadn't given HRT much thought until my GP suggested HRT cream.

I started noticing the dryness last year. My husband and I had improvised on occasion in the past, but this was different. We tried KY jelly from the chemists, but, well, even several dabs didn't really last. I started to feel raw afterwards and things went from bad to worse. This got to my confidence, I think my husband's too, because he didn't want to hurt me.

Sex was uncomfortable, but it was also like I was losing part of me. I married young, but things didn't work out. I only married again in my mid-forties. What I have with my husband now has been very special in my life and I was frightened of losing it. However, it never occurred to me to go to the doctor's until I had bad cystitis.

My GP said that the cystitis and vaginal dryness, everything, could be linked to after the menopause and hormone cream or pessaries might help in future. I wasn't sure about using hormones because I never got on with the Pill, the one time I tried it. I had severe nausea at first, which at least wore off, but not the mood swings and depression. I changed to the diaphragm and used that until I got the all-clear after the menopause.

My GP says HRT uses mostly natural hormones compared to the Pill and, anyway, vaginal HRT isn't anywhere as strong as other treatments. Only that means it won't protect my bones, but that wasn't going to worry me. Vaginal HRT comes as little tablets, not much bigger than coffee sweeteners, with an applicator, but I started on a cream, Ovestin.

I can't tell you, the relief was enormous. I don't think you realize how much something like that slowly gets you down. The cream was a bit awkward, though. I thought maybe it would be like KY jelly, only with hormones in it, but you aren't supposed to use it as a lubricant because it can affect your partner! At first, that wasn't really a problem because I wasn't up to much until everything got better, but then it was difficult to know the best time to use it. Last thing before bed didn't seem right and first thing was rather messy. There again, after a couple of weeks you don't use it every day, just twice a week. Later I changed to Vagifem, the little tablets, instead and used them in the mornings, on days one was due.

After a time it felt like Vagifem wasn't working that well any more. Also my GP said I should think about taking a rest from it. I must say she has been very helpful. She explained that your body can get used to it, so it isn't quite as good. Sort of less is more. I had a few months off but I think perhaps I wasn't ready for sex just then, in my mind or my body. I went back to treatment for another three months and am having a real break now. This time I feel I have got my confidence back. I still get some dryness, but it doesn't feel like the end of the world and I know HRT is there if I need it.

Val

I am nearly 55. Around four years ago, I was in Amsterdam for a weekend and did a lot of walking around sightseeing. Late in the afternoon of the first day I became completely exhausted and could hardly stagger out for an evening meal. This feeling persisted for the next few days.

On returning home I trooped off to the GP. He had no suggestions – I looked healthy. After another episode some months later I returned to him, and he suggested I try sucking a sweet, and other helpful ideas. Subsequently I saw another partner in the practice who did blood tests and more blood tests, but nothing was found. He wondered whether I was depressed. I told him that I wasn't depressed, but that having long bouts of exhaustion could be depressing! Then, of course, the miracle HRT was suggested. I was just the right age.

I refused the HRT and had an abdominal scan, where nothing abnormal was detected. I had an appointment with another partner, who also asked if I was depressed, and suggested HRT. Eventually I was sent to an endocrine specialist, who said I was in real need of HRT for the next twenty years and I bowed to his superior knowledge.

I started with Premique Cycle. My hot flushes disappeared but I still had bouts of exhaustion. Blood tests showed a low level of oestrogen, so I was given different tablets which can be prescribed in a stronger dose (Climagest 2 mg). However, this didn't improve my test results [see p. 60] (I have subsequently discovered that a 'low' oestrogen level is normal for my age, if not for someone on HRT). At this point I felt quite good, in fact a bit overactive, and had developed palpitations, while not being cured of my original complaint of periodic exhaustion. I was finally given a patch to wear (Evorel 100) in addition to the Climagest. After seven months of trial and error, I was starting to worry seriously about the quantity of chemicals that were being poured into me.

I was then told of a doctor who belonged to a group of doctors against the abuse of steroid hormones, whom I contacted. I stopped HRT immediately after seeing her, without any ill effects, and was referred for more tests. I was found to be low in magnesium, chromium and zinc, as well as the essential fatty acids omega 6 and omega 3, and my pancreatic endocrine function was only 23 per cent of normal. I also had a leaky gut. I am on a host of supplements to correct these imbalances, as well as a diet to try to eliminate mild candida that was also found.

This is where it stands at the moment. I am not better yet, but do have increased amounts of energy and some optimism has returned to my life. I have been shocked at the readiness of the traditional medical profession to assume that around the age of 50, all ills are due to the menopause directly, and their readiness to try to convince me that HRT does one a lot of good, especially for osteoporosis, and that the only disadvantage is a 'very slight increase in risk of breast cancer', as if that is something that one might be happy with!

This experience has completely altered my confidence in the GPs and others, and although I have some sympathy with their lack of adequate time for each patient, I feel that they have lost sight of what their profession is all about. I could, but won't, go on! What I am sure of is that, although my bouts of exhaustion are still with me, they are not caused BY my menopause, but rather that with the arrival of the menopause, some other situation has come to light.

Denise

About seven years ago, aged 47, I decided to ask my doctor for HRT. I had heard so much about it in magazines and through friends that I felt this wonder drug was for me. I hoped it would cure my hot flushes and give me a new lease of life. Also the risk of osteoporosis is something to be aware of.

I started off with Prempak-C, which left me feeling spaced out, terrible. I was not on it long, I hasten to add. Next I tried Estrapak, which suited me better, so I stayed on it for about four years. The only problem with this kind of HRT was the monthly 'periods' which lasted 8–9 days each month.

After some particularly heavy bleeding, I was referred to a local specialist who discovered I had fibroids, so a D&C was performed. I decided to stop taking the drug. I just stopped straight away, telling my GP that I'd had enough of the long bleeds. He was OK about this, but he didn't suggest that I stop slowly – enter appalling hot flushes which disturb your sleep patterns so badly! I put up with these symptoms for some months, taking calcium supplements and evening primrose oil. However, thirteen months after stopping HRT I started bleeding again and it was surprisingly heavy.

Back to the hospital for investigation and a further D&C. I asked my consultant if I could take a new HRT that I'd read about, which does not make you bleed each month [continuous combined HRT]. This was called Kliofem and it was relatively new on the market. He said that I needed to be through the menopause before taking it. So he suggested I go back on Estrapak until I was 53 and thus through the menopause, which I did until my birthday last October.

Enter Kliofem! Away went the night sweats and hot flushes and, if I'm honest, mood swings and irritability. Also, there was no bleed. WRONG! There I was – I had been looking forward to our Christmas treat, a long weekend at a stately home health club, and had packed my bag with gym stuff and swimming cozzie for an invigorating weekend. We'd just arrived, unpacked and settled in, when I went to the toilet, and shock, horror, I was bleeding. I had no sanitary protection with me and although the toilets had facilities, I could only use towels, not tampons (because of a tilted womb). Out went the swimming.

I bled for 45 days in all, but it was the week over New Year which was the most terrifying.* On New Year's Eve I was passing large clots so I went to bed, thinking lying down might do the trick. I got up the following day and had to wear pads and sit on towels to stop me soiling the furniture. Every five or ten minutes I would feel these clots dropping down into my vagina and had to put my hand between my legs until I reached the toilet. It was horrendous, I used nearly 40 pads that day.

I made an appointment to see the doctor as soon as they opened after the holidays and he advised me to stop taking the drug, which I did. It took another two weeks before I finally stopped bleeding, it was like a nightmare. So now I don't take anything. I told my doctor I want to be in control of my body, so I am back on the supplements I took before.

However, my hot flushes have crept back and I now have full-blown menopausal symptoms, which are really getting me down. I keep thinking of going back on Estrapak, but then I think about the monthly bleeds and change my mind.

Ingrid

I suppose in a way I looked forward to the menopause. My periods started when I was ten. I flooded at my aunt's house and had to tell her. I remember I was so embarrassed. After that it was monthly hot

---

* The lining of the womb had built up too much while Denise was on Kliofem. Unexpected bleeding can be a problem on continuous combined HRT if women are not sufficiently beyond the menopause.

water bottles and, later, sitting exams dosed up on aspirin. As for PMT – Pretty Miserable Time. So imagine my surprise when my periods petered out last year with not much more than the odd hot flush and I realized I'd 'done it'! Could this be me? Maybe there was a God after all.

I think, in the end, for me the menopause has been about getting older. In your thirties you begin to notice teenagers, how young their skin looks, the gloss on their hair. There is another generation coming along. I remember when I started employing staff in the department (data processing) and realized I could run the team as long as I didn't let on that I could remember when the pocket calculator was invented! But then, just when you think you're getting ahead at work, your hairdresser tactfully suggests you might think about colouring your hair (I gave in) and the skin on your neck shows signs of crepe.

I had my two children late, but they grow up so quickly. My youngest has just started her periods. She's been OK – so far hasn't taken after Mum, at least, not on that score. I think the idea of the menopause being a transition like puberty is helpful. I think of it as a new season in my life, moving from summer to autumn. The menopause is a change and, as you change, that means you leave things behind and gain new ones. Of *course*, I wish I had her skin, but I cannot seriously imagine going through all that painful growing up again! I am happy to be older and – somewhat – wiser.

Though ageing is not easy for women in our society – when did you last see an older woman on the cover of a magazine? Women are taught to make themselves attractive to men and they know that is going to be harder as they get older. Look at all those skin creams and, of course, HRT. An older friend of mine has taken it for about eight years now. She says she started it because her mother had osteoporosis, but I wonder sometimes. It is more acceptable to say that, isn't it? She was very attractive when she was younger and it must be tempting to take something that is supposed to help you keep your looks, even if she'd never admit that that was the reason.

Mind you, I can't pretend that it is easy to age gracefully. But sometimes I think people go too far the other way on this. I like the idea of being 'wise' as well as 'wizened', but I'm not sure that the feminist idea of celebrating the 'crone' is that helpful to most women. Perhaps we should be prepared to accept ageing and what that brings and not feel like second-class citizens or that we have to take hormones to restore our youth or keep us attractive to men. Only now the idea of the crone and reclaiming older women's power has become a commercial gimmick like everything else.

I think the feminist idea that the natural menopause is being turned into an illness is right, though. Next thing ageing itself will be seen as a disease. Isn't it amazing how drug companies use the media to advertise their products even though direct advertising of prescribed medicines to patients is not allowed? Funny how we all know about a certain drug for impotent men now, isn't it? It reminded me of when pop records got banned and then went straight to Number 1. Then there is this new 'designer' HRT in several women's magazines I read. They think it won't have the same risk of breast cancer. I even heard an advertising man interviewed on the radio about these new 'lifestyle' drugs – Viagra, HRT and another one for weight loss. He said they know patient groups and women's magazines want to keep us informed, so his job is to turn a new drug into a news story! I couldn't believe that he came right out and said that, like we are all really stupid.

4

HORMONE REPLACEMENT THERAPY

'I have found all the way along this road that I would have liked more information on the drugs I was being asked to take. I like to know what I am taking, how it works in my body and what side-effects it may cause – I need to feel happy with it.'

KATE

Increasing numbers of women are being offered hormone replacement therapy (HRT) in some shape or form. This chapter looks at what women are being asked to take and why. It shows women how to decipher what is in a packet of HRT and discusses the vexed question of what counts as a natural hormone. It goes on to describe the main side-effects and what can be done to reduce them. Finally the chapter looks at testosterone therapy and whether the new 'designer' oestrogens will revolutionize HRT.

What is HRT?

Hormone replacement therapy is the name given to drugs that provide forms of oestrogen alone or *combined* drugs that provide forms of oestrogen *and* progesterone. The active ingredients are either hormones like those found in the body or related compounds. They may be so-called natural or synthetic hormones. In general, the doses used in HRT provide hormone levels that are lower than those during the menstrual cycle (although see page 219).

Oestrogens are used in HRT to alleviate menopausal symptoms such as hot flushes, night sweats and vaginal dryness (Figure 4.1).

Doctors also recommend long-term therapy to reduce the risks of heart disease and osteoporosis in later life. These problems are thought to be due to the fall in oestrogen levels after the menopause, which leads to a state of 'oestrogen deficiency'. By definition, this state can be remedied by 'replacement' therapy. However, the view that post-menopausal women are oestrogen deficient is controversial. Opponents argue that the fall in oestrogen at this time of life is a normal state of affairs and that women's hormones do not need replacing as such because they are not *missing*. Only younger women who lack oestrogen may need 'replacement'. This debate is explored further in Chapter 9.

Progesterone also falls during the menopause, but, in general, doctors do not regard menopausal women as 'progesterone deficient' (although see Chapter 11). Instead, synthetic forms of progesterone (progest*ogens*) are included in HRT to protect women from the increased risk of endometrial cancer if oestrogen is used on its own (unopposed). The extra risk of endometrial cancer became evident during the controversial early history of HRT when women were given oestrogen therapy before its effects were better understood (some feel little has changed, Chapter 9). The result was that more women developed endometrial cancer than would have done if they had not been taking hormones. Belatedly doctors realized that taking oestrogen alone can overstimulate the lining of the womb and double the risk of endometrial cancer.

In the UK, oestrogen-only HRT is given to women who do not have a womb, either because of a hysterectomy or perhaps because they were born without one. British women who have wombs are prescribed combined HRT, either in a pre-packaged form or according to guidelines on the 'safe' doses of different progestogens, i.e. doses that will 'oppose' standard measures of oestrogen. In the USA, oestrogen-only therapy (ERT – oestrogen is spelled 'estrogen' in the States) is widely used and the risk of endometrial cancer is managed by monitoring women with wombs for warning signs of overstimulation (e.g. by taking regular biopsies of the lining of the womb).

This difference can seem rather odd. One reason American doctors

Figure 4.1 HRT and menopausal symptoms

Studies have shown that HRT can alleviate hot flushes and night sweats (although the effect of 'dummy' pills can be important, see page 207). Some women find their symptoms improve quickly, but for others relief takes several weeks of treatment. Women who do not benefit within the first few months may need a larger dose or a different type of HRT. In particular, younger women can need higher doses than those usually prescribed for women in the natural menopause.[1] Also, occasionally women have trouble absorbing hormones in tablet form.

HRT can help vaginal dryness, either when used in the vagina (e.g. as a vaginal tablet or cream) or when taken bodily (e.g. as a tablet, skin patch or implant). This can make a big difference to women who suffer painful or burning symptoms of dryness (see Maureen, Chapter 3) or who get a discharge or bleeding after intercourse.

Urinary incontinence can be another distressing problem for post-menopausal women. Doctors thought that this was due to oestrogen deficiency, but research has shown that this is not the case as such.[2] Furthermore, HRT is not a useful treatment. However, women who develop recurrent cystitis after the menopause can benefit from vaginal HRT (which is absorbed into the surrounding area).[3]

HRT can be prescribed in the hope of relieving complaints such as forgetfulness, tiredness and depression. However, the evidence that HRT can resolve these problems is mixed and there is a danger that other medical causes may be overlooked simply because a woman is in her menopause. Equally such complaints may be due to other aspects of life or part of ageing itself. This does not make them any less distressing for the women concerned, but it does mean that HRT is not the answer.

prefer to prescribe oestrogen-only is because most of the research over the years has been done on this type of HRT (particularly the long-established brand Premarin). It is not yet clear whether adding a progestogen alters the long-term risks and benefits. This uncertainty means that British doctors may only recommend lengthy use of combined HRT to post-menopausal women who have several risk factors for osteoporosis and are therefore more likely to benefit. In contrast, doctors have no hesitation about prescribing long-term combined HRT to women who lose their hormones at an early age since this itself is a risk factor for osteoporosis and heart disease.

Combined HRT involves taking two hormones in a monthly pattern that mimics the menstrual cycle and leads to regular 'periods' in 90 per cent of women.[4] Doctors describe these periods as 'withdrawal bleeds'. Withdrawal bleeds take place because the womb's lining has grown in response to the oestrogen in HRT and then is shed. Having 'periods' may cheer younger women who want some sense of normality, but it can be very unwelcome to women after the natural menopause and many give up HRT for this reason.

Drugs companies have responded to this 'drop-out' by developing newer forms of combined HRT for post-menopausal women which are said to be 'bleed free'. These brands are known as *continuous* combined HRT because they do not have to be taken in a monthly pattern. This type of HRT is still experimental and little research has been done on its longer-term risks and benefits. Tibolone (Livial) is a different type of drug that can be used as 'bleed-free' HRT. Tibolone has been around for many years, but has not been widely used or studied in large groups of women compared to other kinds of HRT.

Women may find that they are offered testosterone as an addition to their HRT, especially if they have had their ovaries removed. Testosterone replacement therapy is thought to enhance libido, although again its use is largely experimental. The same note of caution applies to the new 'designer' oestrogens (SERMs) since little is known about long-term use.

To summarize, at present HRT refers to either a preparation of oestrogen-only or a combination of hormones. A combination can be taken in a monthly pattern with periods or, sometimes, continuously to avoid bleeding. Once it is clear which type of HRT is appropriate, women may be offered a choice of pills, skin patches, implants, body gels, etc. These different forms of HRT are described in detail in Chapter 10. Occasionally younger women who lack hormones are offered the contraceptive pill as HRT.

Deciphering the Ingredients

The body has three types of oestrogen (17-beta-oestradiol, oestrone and oestriol) and one kind of progesterone. However, these hormones may not be among the ingredients listed on a packet of HRT. Some of the reasons for this are commercial; others are to do with what happens to a drug inside the body. Understanding a bit more about this can help to unravel some of the arguments about the ingredients in HRT, including whether they are natural or synthetic. It can also help to explain what doctors mean when they say that certain types of HRT 'bypass' the liver.

To work, a drug must have active ingredients that can enter the body and reach the place where help is wanted. These ingredients may reach their destination unchanged or be chemically converted by the body into their active form somewhere along the way. A drug must have a therapeutic effect before being broken down or expelled by the body and, preferably, without causing too many unwanted effects elsewhere, i.e. *side*-effects. All this is true whether the drug is a conventional medicine or, say, a herbal remedy (although herbal remedies contain numerous substances in varying amounts and the active ingredients are often unknown, see Chapter 12).

Drugs are so familiar that their task can appear simple. However, swallowing a tablet only takes it inside the stomach, a place full of acids and enzymes that are good at breaking down substances because this is how they turn food into serviceable molecules for the body. To be effective, the relevant drug ingredients must survive in a useful form. Then, when they move on from the stomach, they must be able to pass through the walls of the gut into the bloodstream. The lining of the gut is a kind of 'border control' or filter that only allows certain molecules to enter the blood vessels that run alongside. Enough of the drug's ingredients must get through the lining in an active form to provide an effective dose. Otherwise the drug will continue out of the body in the faeces having done nothing beneficial.

Once the drug is through the lining of the gut, it must be able to dissolve in the bloodstream (i.e. be soluble in water) or hitch a ride with another molecule. However, before it can be ferried to its destination, it has to survive a journey through the liver. The liver has several roles in the body including sorting out unwanted or redundant substances. The blood vessels surrounding the small intestine take blood directly to the liver for sorting before it enters the main circulation. This is known as the 'first pass' through the liver. It is also what doctors are talking about when they say that one of the disadvantages of oral HRT is that it does not bypass the liver. Often a dose taken by mouth has to be relatively high to compensate for the fact that the liver will destroy much of it at this first hurdle.

The remaining dose will pass into the main circulation which visits the whole body. If the active ingredient is identical to a hormone produced by the body, then it can fit the relevant receptors and unlock change (see Chapter 2). However, it can also unlock change if it is a related molecule that acts as a skeleton key. In this case, the drug will have hormone-like effects. The length of time a drug remains active depends on how well it survives the 'second pass' through the liver. All the blood in the body circulates through the liver every five minutes so that unwanted substances (usually waste from cells rather than drugs) can be cleared. A lot of these substances are broken down by the liver and sent back into the gut to be expelled from the body. They may also be cleared from the blood by the kidneys and passed into the urine. This is why on-going medical conditions need repeated drug treatment (although this can bring its own problems).

The barriers described above explain why one may not be able to take a hormone by swallowing it. Often one has to take a related substance that will survive the hazards of the gut and be converted into the required hormone or something similar enough. For example, in the past only oestriol could be taken orally. Oestradiol, the strongest type of oestrogen, does not get through the gut lining very well because it is not very soluble in water. However, now it has been produced in a micronized (miniaturized) form that the gut can absorb. Other tablets use related oestrogen compounds, such as oestradiol valerate or piperazine oestrone sulphate, to solve this problem. The body chemically converts many of these substances into oestrone by the time they reach the bloodstream.[5] That is, the main active ingredient that appears in the blood after taking many of the different oestrogen compounds in HRT tablets is actually the *same*.

Swallowing progesterone has drawbacks too. Although some of it will reach the bloodstream this way, the body is so good at dismantling progesterone to make other substances that the dose may not get a chance to work. This is one of the pragmatic reasons why HRT tablets often contain related compounds known as progest*ogens* (UK) or progest*ins* (USA). These substances have had some of their molecular side chains altered so that they are dismantled less readily by the liver and have time to act on the progesterone receptors, causing progesterone-like effects. Of course, there are also commercial reasons for producing progestogens, since the 'copyright' for their structures belongs to the drug company rather than Nature.

Sometimes the gut and 'first pass' through the liver can be avoided by introducing a drug into the body in another way. Drugs can be injected just below the skin or absorbed directly into the circulation from creams, gels or skin patches. They can also reach the bloodstream through the lining of the vagina, anus or nose. Vaginal rings, pessaries or creams, anal suppositories, nasal sprays – the list is lengthy and varied. In some cases the method of delivering the hormone has the 'copyright' (e.g. the type of patch adhesive) and so a natural hormone may be used. However, these non-oral methods won't work for every drug. For example, it may be difficult to produce a liquid form that can be injected safely. Equally the active ingredient may not be absorbed sufficiently through the skin or other body surfaces.

Oestradiol lends itself to numerous non-oral types of HRT because it dissolves in alcohol and is then absorbed readily by the skin or through the vaginal lining. It is used widely in patches and gels, subcutaneous implants, vaginal rings, pessaries and creams. As these methods bypass the effects of the gut and liver, they can use smaller doses of oestradiol (micrograms, (μg or mcg), rather than milligrams, mg, found in tablets) to provide equivalent blood levels. Tablets or injections of progesterone tend to have a brief effect, but progesterone is available as anal suppositories, vaginal gels or, controversially, in alternative skin creams.

Knowing what happens to HRT in the body can help doctors work out what to measure to check whether it has 'arrived'. This may not be as simple as it sounds. For example, the standard 'oestrogen' blood test measures oestradiol. That can be rather meaningless if used to judge the many tablets whose ingredients are converted largely to oestrone in the bloodstream. However, the test *can* be used to monitor non-tablet forms of HRT, where oestradiol reaches the bloodstream intact. That said, even the results of tests in women taking the same dose of the same HRT can vary widely because their bodies absorb and break down the drug at different speeds. There are similar pitfalls when it comes to measuring the effects of natural progesterone.

Given the body's apparent obstacle course, it can seem surprising that drugs ever work! But, obviously, drugs can and *do* have powerful effects and HRT is no exception. Some women are happy to leave the details of a drug like HRT to their doctors; others have such awful menopausal symptoms that, understandably, they just want something that makes them feel better. However, many women want to know what they are being asked to take and prefer the idea of natural hormones. This begs the question of what counts as a natural hormone (assuming that it is natural to take hormones at all).

Natural or Synthetic?

The word 'natural' has been described as an advertiser's dream, second only to the word 'new'. It is a word that matters and not least when it comes to HRT. But what does it mean? If natural means 'as in nature', then this might mean ingredients from a natural source and/or hormones like those found in the body. But what if substances identical to those found in nature can be synthesized and the body reacts to them as if they are the real thing? Furthermore, what if *related* substances can be produced from a natural source that can also unlock hormone receptors?

The idea that natural hormones are those found in the body is a useful anchor in this debate. In this case, there are three natural oestrogens (17-beta-oestradiol, oestrone, oestriol) and one natural progesterone. However, as explained in the previous section, one might need to take a related compound to produce one of these hormones in the body. For example, HRT tablets can contain oestrogen compounds that are not found in the body, but are largely converted into oestrone – which *is*. Doctors tend to describe such compounds as natural oestrogens. Is this stretching the definition?

A similar question arises with HRT that contains 'conjugated equine oestrogens'. These are a mixture of 50–65 per cent oestrone sulphate and the horse oestrogen equilin sulphate. Women's bodies convert the first substance to oestrone and the second to equilin. Here, the yardstick that doctors use to conclude that equilin is 'natural' is its structural similarity to human oestrogens and its capacity to act on relevant receptors. For example, equilin has one chemical link that is slightly different and occurs in 'mirror' forms.[6] But, as described in Chapter 2, slight differences can have more than a slight effect. The liver finds it harder to break down equilin and so it lasts longer in the body. Researchers do not know whether this matters. It may be the reason for certain side-effects; it may also cause beneficial changes in lipoproteins.[7]

Conjugated equine oestrogens come from a natural source, *pregnant mares' urine* (hence the brand name Premarin, also Prempak-C, etc.). However, this does not appeal to some women and others object to horses being farmed for this purpose (see More Help). This may be one of the reasons why patient leaflets for other brands are often quick to point out that they are made from soy beans or cacti, although they tend not to add that this means that the active ingredients have been *synthesized* in a laboratory from *related* plant substances. For

Basic steroid structure

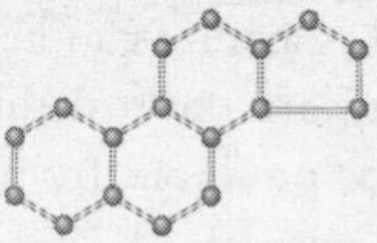

Natural oestrogens

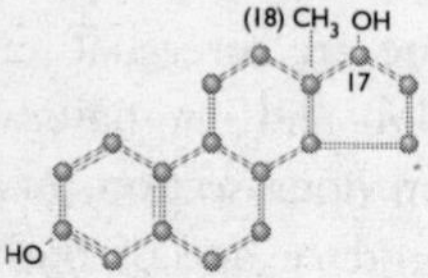

Oestradiol 17β

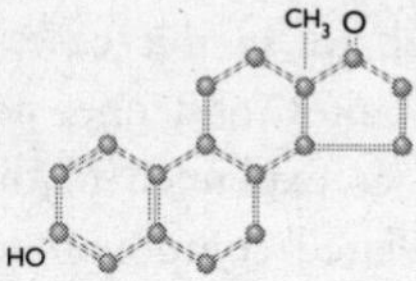

Oestrone

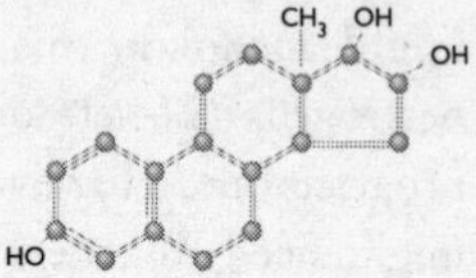

Oestriol

Synthetic oestrogens

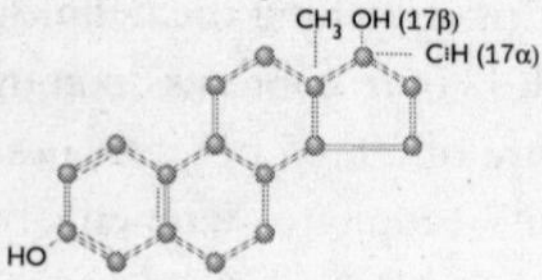

Ethinyl oestradiol

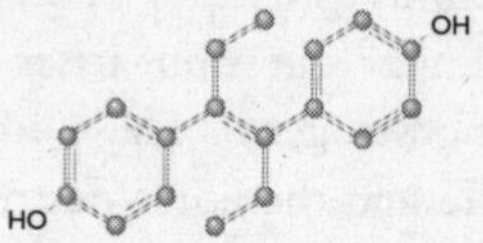

Diethylstilbestrol (DES)*

Phytoestrogens

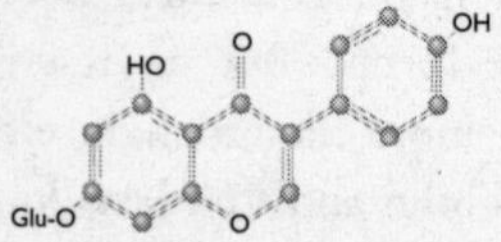

Genistin (isoflavone glucoside)*
(e.g. in soy foods)

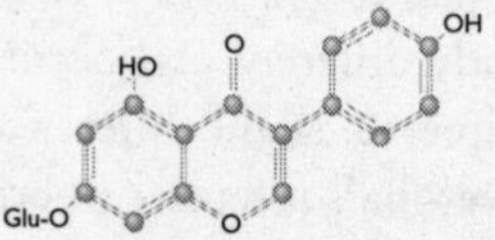

Daidzin (isoflavone glucoside)*
(e.g. in soy foods)

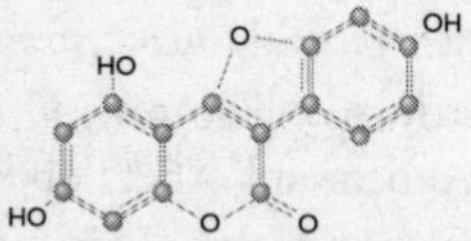

Coumestrol* (e.g. in traditional
Chinese medicine)

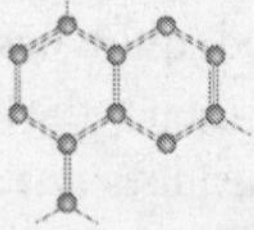

Diterpene* (sclareol in
clary sage essential oil
is a diterpenic alcohol)

*Non–steroid structures

Figure 4.2 Spot the difference

example, the natural hormone oestradiol, so widely used in certain tablets, skin patches, gels, implants and vaginal creams, is synthesized. Even the natural progesterone in the alternative skin creams that have provoked so much interest is made in the lab.

Does this matter? Doctors who support the use of natural oestradiol would say 'no' because the hormone produced is identical to that found in the body. A similar argument is advanced by supporters of natural progesterone. However, others argue that women are better off trying to relieve menopausal symptoms with natural 'plant oestrogens' such as those found in soy foods (phytoestrogens, see Chapter 12). This sounds tempting because surely they are natural in every sense? Yet even here the question is fraught. For example, one American doctor has been keen to point out that some of the phytoestrogens that women are embracing are not 'exactly natural' when measured with the yard-stick of structural similarity. He comments that the horse oestrogen equilin is much closer in structure to human oestrogens than many plant oestrogens, which do not have 'steroid' rings (see Figure 4.2).[8]

Doctors use the term 'synthetic oestrogen' for compounds such as ethinyl oestradiol, mestranol and dienoestrol because the body cannot convert them into substances like those found in the body. This sounds undesirable and it is in some ways. Yet, paradoxically, it can also be the reason why these drugs work. For example, the contraceptive pill uses ethinyl oestradiol because its structural differences from natural oestradiol mean that it can be taken by mouth and is demolished by the liver far less easily. As a result, even small doses are potent enough to prevent pregnancy, unlike HRT, which relies on natural oestrogens and is *not* contraceptive.

All the substances in Figure 4.2 can act in the body. However, they can have very different effects. For example, ethinyl oestradiol is far more potent than natural oestradiol. Also, diethylstilbestrol (DES) may look oddly similar to the oestrogenic substances found in soy foods (genistin and daidzin), but DES is a controversial synthetic oestrogen that was given to prevent miscarriage until the mid 1970s when it was realized, belatedly, that it led to congenital abnormalities.

Ethinyl oestradiol can be used as hormone replacement because it acts on the same oestrogen receptors as HRT. It may be prescribed alone or in the form of the contraceptive pill for younger women who lack hormones. However, its long-term use is controversial (see pages 114 and 146) and the natural oestrogens already described are used more frequently as HRT. In contrast, synthetic forms of progesterone are almost standard in conventional HRT.

The term progest*ogen* refers to a synthetic compound that is not produced by the body, but can act as a skeleton key on progesterone receptors. Often such compounds are described rather loosely as progesterone, which is not the case. However, the distinction begins to blur when one has to consider the progestogen called dydrogesterone. By the time dydrogesterone reaches the receptors the body has converted it to the 'real' thing. Ironically no one describes this as natural progesterone (unlike oestrogenic compounds, which are described as natural oestrogens when they are converted by the body into their natural counterparts).

The debate about natural and synthetic hormones is not just about the ingredients used; it is also about the methods of delivering the hormone. For example, sometimes oestradiol skin patches and implants are described as more 'physiological' (body-like) because they trickle hormone into the body. This contrasts with the wave of hormone caused by taking a tablet. Indeed, some doctors say that the disadvantage of HRT tablets is not so much the 'first pass' through the liver, but that the liver gets the whole daily dose in one go.[9] Non-oral HRT is also said to be more physiological because it leads to a 'body-like' ratio of oestradiol and oestrone in the bloodstream. All this sounds comforting because 'physiological' doses or delivery appear to be more natural. However, here 'natural' means natural to a body before the menopause. This returns to the question of whether it is natural to take hormones after the natural menopause, even if one does this in a more physiological way. In the end, it is a personal decision.

Side-effects

The return of 'periods', weight gain and the risk of breast cancer are the problems associated with taking HRT that worry women the most. The risk of breast cancer is compared with the possible benefits of HRT in Chapter 5. The main side-effects of HRT are given in Figure 4.3. Contraindications for HRT are given in Figure 4.4.

Figure 4.3 Main side-effects of HRT

Oestrogens

Nausea

Fluid retention

Breast tenderness/enlargement/nipple sensitivity

Headaches

Weight gain

C19 progestogens (e.g. norethisterone, norgestrel and levonorgestrel)

'Premenstrual tension'

Bloating

Breast tenderness

Mood swings

Depression

Weight gain

Headaches

Acne

C21 progestogens (e.g. medroxyprogesterone acetate (MPA) or dydrogesterone)

Said to be few compared to C19s

Miscellaneous

Occasional visual disturbances, possible trouble wearing contact lenses due to changes in the shape of the eye

Due to delivery method

- Gastrointestinal upsets due to tablets
- Unexpected spotting or prolonged bleeding on continuous combined HRT if used by younger women or those who are not far enough beyond the menopause
- Skin irritation due to patches
- Tiny scars due to implants; occasional wound infections or resurfacing of the implant
- Unwanted growth of lining of the womb (endometrial hyperplasia) if vaginal HRT is used in high doses or long-term unopposed by a progestogen
- Side-effects in sexual partners if vaginal HRT is used as sexual lubricant

Surveys have shown that 'withdrawal bleeds' are the main reason why women do not stay on HRT for long after the natural menopause.[10] Many women feel that such 'periods' are unnatural or just plain inconvenient. In this case, women may wish to try 'bleed-free' HRT, although breakthrough bleeding can be a problem. This is more likely in younger women or women who may not be sufficiently past the menopause.

Women who complain of weight gain on HRT may be greeted with scepticism by their GPs. Doctors can regard overeating and/or lack of exercise as simply the most likely explanation. Alternatively they may point to the redistribution of body fat that can follow the menopause. Specifically women can gain weight round the waist having lost it from their hips and/or bust. This may feel like a weight gain because clothes no longer fit as before. Doctors may also express doubt because a three-year clinical trial found that menopausal women on HRT put on *less* weight than those on placebos.[11] The researchers suggested that the weight gain in women taking placebos was age-related. Among the women taking HRT, those on oestrogen-only therapy put on less weight than those on combined HRT. However, as other doctors acknowledge, this study reports differences between the averages for large groups of women and does not provide information about individual cases. Some women may have put on a lot of weight without affecting the average for their group because this was not a common enough experience. A British doctor has commented that in her clinical experience some patients do seem to put on a 'startling' amount of weight on HRT.[12] She suggests various options, including trying a different type of HRT, using diuretics to reduce fluid retention or organizing a temporary 'time out' from HRT. Women who suffer this problem can be tempted to take such 'time out' anyway, perhaps especially if they are disillusioned by their doctor's response (see Susan, Chapter 7). However, if they do so without support and advice, they can suffer severe withdrawal symptoms. Also, younger women who vote with their feet, albeit for very understandable reasons, are in a double bind: they run a greater risk of osteoporosis and heart disease than older women if they abandon treatment completely.

Sometimes women find that side-effects improve on a different type of HRT because the ingredients or delivery method of a particular brand did not agree with them. For example, oestrogens taken as tablets can cause nausea at first. Although it tends to wear off, it can be a persistent – and debilitating – problem. Nausea may be due to a problem with absorption, in which case it can be managed by taking the tablets during meal-times or last thing at night.[13] If nausea is a response to tablets containing synthetic ethinyl oestradiol or high doses of natural oestrogen, then starting on a low dose and building up may help. Otherwise it may be best to switch away from the synthetic oestrogen and/or the tablets to, say, skin patches.

Oestrogens are also associated with breast tenderness. Women can find this alarming because it is an unwelcome reminder that HRT can stimulate breast tissue. This is an understandable worry, but breast tenderness is not associated with breast cancer. Usually this side-effect wears off after the early months of treatment. That said, it can be a very uncomfortable, if not painful, experience until it does! Some women find that cutting out tea and coffee helps, as may sleeping in a sports bra. Alternatively sufficient doses of evening primrose oil (EPO) can make a difference.

Figure 4.4 Contraindications for HRT

Looking at the patient information leaflet which comes with HRT can be worrying because so many contraindications (reasons for not taking it) are listed. To make matters worse, some researchers do not agree with these lists, arguing that they are overcautious,[14] and prescribing guidelines for doctors acknowledge that the evidence for some of these contra-indications is limited.[15] Anyone in doubt after reading this list is advised to talk to their doctor, especially if they are on HRT and do not receive check-ups.

There is general agreement that HRT is not recommended in the following cases:

- oestrogen-dependent cancers such as breast
  cancer or endometrial cancer (lining of the womb)
- severe active liver disease
- active thrombosis (blood clot) disorders
- during breastfeeding

Current guidelines also say that HRT must be prescribed with caution in cases where it may pose an additional risk or exacerbate the condition:

- a strong family history of breast cancer
- previous benign breast lumps
- history of blood clots (thrombosis)
- endometriosis or fibroids (benign
  oestrogen-dependent conditions)
- gallstones
- porphyria
- migraines or similar headaches

Drug company leaflets also advise women to check with their doctors if they have the following conditions but, as described above, there is some debate about whether there is enough evidence to be cautious about prescribing HRT in these cases:

- epilepsy
- high blood pressure
- asthma
- melanoma
- multiple sclerosis
- thyrotoxicosis
- otosclerosis
- systemic lupus erythematosus

Difficulties can arise for women with epilepsy, asthma and those taking thyroxine because of interactions between HRT and other medication.[16]

Many of the other common side-effects are caused by the progestogens in combined HRT. Doctors may suggest reducing the dose (although this should be within safe limits to protect against the risk of endometrial cancer). If this does not help, then women may benefit from changing to another group of progestogens. Drug-company chemists make progestogens in two general forms. The C19 family, which is more closely related to testosterone, has a reputation for side-effects, such as feeling bloated, 'premenstrual tension', depression, headaches and acne. If women have problems with one C19 progestogen, then they are unlikely to improve on a brand containing another. However, they may feel better on HRT that uses a newer C21 progestogen. That said, drug companies have been trying to develop new forms of the C19 progestogens with fewer side-effects (e.g. gestodene). These substances have appeared in the contraceptive pill and may become part of HRT. Another option is to try skin patches of combined HRT (e.g. Estracombi, Nuvelle TS, Evorelsequi), which avoid the 'first pass' through the liver and therefore require less progestogen to deliver an effective dose.

Other non-oral forms of progesterone are being developed. These could be used as part of combined HRT and prove to have fewer side-effects for the reason above. For example, there is an IUD (intrauterine device) that releases progestogen and a vaginal gel which contains natural progesterone (Crinone). The vaginal gel is not to be confused with the 'alternative' natural progesterone skin cream that has attracted interest and controversy. The gel uses a higher dose of natural progesterone, one which, an early study indicates, is protective judging by its effects on the lining of the womb.[17] The safety of using 'alternative' natural progesterone skin creams with oestrogen as combined HRT is unknown. However, advocates argue that this is not an issue with the cream because it relieves menopausal symptoms by using body-like doses of natural progesterone without any need for oestrogen. At this stage, all these options are highly experimental.

Testosterone

Testosterone has been described as the 'hormone of desire'[18] – in both sexes – and testosterone replacement therapy is exciting considerable interest as a result. However, the idea that testosterone can affect women's libido is not new. Synthetic forms of testosterone were produced in the late 1930s and used during the 1940s to treat women with oestrogen-dependent cancers.[19] It was reported then that these drugs could increase libido, but they also caused a range of unwelcome side-effects such as acne, hirsutism (hairiness), voice deepening and enlargement of the clitoris. In retrospect, these side-effects are not surprising given the large doses that women were given.

Interest in testosterone therapy has revived since then. Now it is suggested that women can suffer from testosterone deficiency after the menopause as well as lack of oestrogen. It is true that testosterone levels change, but it is less clear whether this results in a state of deficiency. During the menstrual cycle testosterone levels show slight but regular variations, rising during ovulation and again in the second half. The purpose of this is unknown, although one suggestion is that the mid-cycle peak promotes libido at a time when sexual intercourse is more likely to result in pregnancy. Testosterone and related androgen hormones begin to fall in the years before the menopause and some researchers have commented that this may account for symptoms such as lack of energy, lower sex drive and reduction in bone mass.[20] They argue that this gradual overall fall is one of the reasons why it is difficult to show a clear relationship between testosterone levels and symptoms of testosterone deficiency. Instead, they point to studies of testosterone therapy in women who have had their ovaries removed.

Women's testosterone levels drop by 50 per cent after oophorectomy (testosterone is still made elsewhere in the body). In contrast, the fall after the natural menopause is only about 20 per cent because the ovaries continue some androgen production. Women can suffer from lack of libido after surgery in spite of taking oestrogen-only HRT to combat vaginal dryness, and doctors have found that adding testosterone appears to improve this problem. Nevertheless, there have been only a few small placebo-controlled studies of testosterone HRT. Their findings suggest that it may increase women's reported arousal but not necessarily their sexual activity. Some researchers have also questioned the merits of these studies because of the doses used.[21] Modern doses are far lower than those prescribed 50 years ago, but there is still a debate about the risk of unwanted side-effects. Some doctors advocate physiological doses of testosterone to avoid this risk; others question whether such low doses can be effective. These issues are explored in more detail in Chapters 8 and 10.

In short, the biochemistry of testosterone is very complicated because testosterone is produced by more than one part of the body and converted from and to related hormones. There are also interactions between testosterone and oestrogen that may affect women's sensitivity. For example, one group of researchers have noted that oestrogen-only HRT may reduce the availability of what is known as free testosterone and that this could lead to symptoms of testosterone deficiency.[22]

It may be some time before the questions have been answered. What is the most advisable dose of testosterone HRT given the risk of side-effects? How long should treatment last? What are the long-term risks and benefits? At present, limited evidence suggests that testosterone therapy may help women who have had their ovaries removed. This may also apply to women born without ovaries (although perhaps not those who are completely androgen insensitive, see Chapter 6). The position is less clear for women who have a natural or premature menopause and experience a gradual change in their testosterone levels.

According to some doctors, testosterone deficiency could become a general problem as more women live longer and testosterone HRT could become a way of 'protecting quality of life'.[23] Elsewhere testosterone deficiency has been criticized as another example of 'popular expectations and commercial motives helping to define new medical "disorders"'.[24] This debate is discussed more widely in Chapter 9.

'Designer' Oestrogens (SERMs)

'Designer' oestrogens have attracted a lot of interest among researchers because they appear to offer a way round women's fears of developing breast cancer as a result of taking HRT.[25] Despite their popular name, 'designer' oestrogens are not forms of oestrogen such as those used in conventional HRT. Instead, they are what is known technically as *s*elective *e*strogen-*r*eceptor *m*odulators (SERMs).

The SERM family of drugs is related to tamoxifen, which is used to treat breast cancer because it *blocks* the effect of women's own oestrogen on breast tissue. However, tamoxifen also *acts like* oestrogen in other areas of the body, e.g. the bones. That is, unlike conventional HRT, it can act *selectively*, blocking some oestrogen receptors and stimulating others. Researchers realized that substances that were oestrogen-*like* in some parts of the body – but *not* breast tissue – might reduce women's risk of osteoporosis without increasing their risk of breast cancer.

A form of HRT that avoids any extra risk of breast cancer sounds promising and the first of these drugs, raloxifene (Evista), is available already on prescription in the UK and USA. Its arrival has been greeted with great enthusiasm by some doctors, who regard it as shifting the goalposts of the whole HRT debate. Others are more cautious, noting its limitations – not least that it is licensed for the prevention of osteoporosis only. Raloxifene does not relieve hot flushes.

This seems somewhat ironic for a 'designer' oestrogen, especially when one considers that menopausal women tend to seek treatment for hot flushes, if they seek treatment at all. Perhaps new SERMs will be produced that do all the 'right' things. Until then, women may find that they are offered old-fashioned HRT during the menopause followed by preventive treatment for osteoporosis with a SERM. This option is experimental at present and it will be some time before there is any data on the long-term risks and benefits of SERMs.

5

HEART DISEASE, OSTEOPOROSIS
AND BREAST CANCER

*'Most medical interventions . . . do not offer a certain cure in
an otherwise hopeless situation.'*[1]

Increasingly women are told that HRT is the way to better hearts
and bones. Yet women are wary of any extra risk of breast cancer.
Where does the balance lie? This chapter looks at what doctors
regard as the major benefits of HRT versus women's concerns.
It starts with a brief guide to the pitfalls of risk data. Then it takes
each disease in turn, asking what oestrogen has to do with it and
how HRT may alter the chances of developing the problem. In
doing so, it shows how the odds depend on *when* women lose their
hormones.

Getting to Grips with Risk

Much of this chapter is about one's risks of developing certain diseases
and how HRT could affect the odds. New research may change the
estimates and shift the equation, but women will still be faced with
trying to understand what is being said – by doctors and the media
– and how this relates to them.

There are several things to watch for when risks are quoted.
For example, what time period do they refer to? Take the following
information: women have a 23 per cent lifetime risk of dying from
heart disease (see Figure 5.1). Here, one is being given a *lifetime*
risk. Twenty-three out of every 100 women will die for this reason.

The remaining 77 in every 100 will die of something else. Yet common sense says that a baby girl and a 50-year-old woman have different risks over their *remaining* lifetime. So while both have the 23 per cent lifetime risk, the woman having survived 50 years without dying from childhood illness, car accident, etc., now has a 31 per cent risk of fatal heart disease during her remaining life.

The value of 31 per cent for a 50-year-old woman is less than that given in Figure 5.1. This is because the second set of data refers to the chances of *having* a disease rather than dying from it. This is another piece of information to watch out for because, obviously, the chances of having a disease are not necessarily the same as the chances of dying from it.

Increases or decreases in risk may be given as percentages or fractions. For example, a common message is that 'HRT can reduce the risk of a hip fracture by about 30 per cent and a spine fracture by about 50 per cent.'[2] Perhaps it is helpful to think of these as price tags to see what sort of deal is being offered. As shoppers well know, the value of anything off depends on the original price of the goods. Likewise, if HRT halves or doubles the risk of something, one might ask, 'What was the risk in the first place?'

For example, younger women have less risk of breast cancer than older women. Furthermore, young women who lose their hormones have a lower risk of breast cancer than friends their age. Therefore the slight extra risk of breast cancer linked with taking long-term HRT is not thought to make much difference to their odds before the age of 50. In contrast, women with the BRCA1 gene have what is known as a very high 'absolute' risk of breast cancer compared to others their age. Therefore the slightly increased risk of breast cancer on HRT could make a big difference to them.

Figure 5.1 Summary of relevant risks and remaining questions

In general, a woman has the following risks during her lifetime:
- 23 per cent risk of *dying* of heart disease
- 4 per cent risk of dying of breast cancer
- 2.5 per cent risk of dying due to an osteoporotic fracture

A woman aged 50 has the following risks in her remaining lifetime:[3]
- 45 per cent risk of *having* heart disease
- 15 per cent risk of having a hip fracture
- 8 per cent risk of having breast cancer

Some women's risks will be higher or lower depending on their other risk factors, including whether they have lacked hormones from an early age.

HRT to reduce the risks of heart disease

- This is still the subject of much debate.
- Starting HRT is *not* advised for women with established heart disease given the results of the HERS study (see page 84).
- HRT is claimed to halve women's risk; the true reduction may be nearer a third.
- Women may only benefit while taking HRT.
- It is not clear whether women using non-oral HRT or those who need to take progestogens benefit to quite the same extent.
- The benefit does not appear to be dose-related.

HRT to reduce the risks of osteoporosis

- HRT can reduce the risk of a hip fracture by 30 per cent and a spinal fracture by 50 per cent.
- Women must be on a sufficient dose (see Figure 10.1, page 214).
- Women may only benefit while taking HRT and for some time thereafter.
- It is not clear for how long women should take HRT after the menopause to reduce later fractures.
- The benefit may be improved by some progestogens.

HRT and the extra risk of breast cancer

- Women are at risk of breast cancer whether they take HRT or not.
- The main risk factor is increasing age.
- Taking HRT can add to a woman's existing risk (see Figure 5.7, page 96).
- The additional risk depends on length of treatment, but not dose.
- After stopping HRT, the extra risk disappears within five years.
- Progestogens do not appear to lower the extra risk (unlike their effect on the extra risk of endometrial cancer).

HRT and the extra risk of endometrial cancer

- Oestrogen therapy increases the risk of endometrial cancer in women with wombs during and after use.
- This extra risk is reduced by 'opposing' oestrogen with a sufficient dose of progestogen.

HRT and the extra risk of thrombosis (blood clots)

- Women have a very small risk of thrombosis whether they take HRT or not.
- Women on HRT have three times this small risk.
- Thrombosis is serious for the few affected because sudden death can result if blood clots lodge in the heart or brain. This is more likely during initial treatment.

The risk of thrombosis provides another example. HRT triples the chances of this happening. Yet most women's existing risk of thrombosis is very low, so doctors do not regard this increased risk as a major reason against treatment. One could say that triple something small is still something small. Which *isn't* to say that the consequences aren't serious – even fatal – for the minority concerned. This is the dilemma.

Sometimes increases and decreases in risk are misinterpreted because of the maths involved. For example, one study estimated that

HRT increased women's risk of breast cancer by 50 per cent. Several journalists misunderstood this result and alarmed women with their conclusions.[4] As mentioned above, women need to ask what their risk is in the first place before deciding how much to worry about a 50 per cent increase. Secondly, one has to sidestep the trap of thinking that a 50 per cent *increase in risk* means that 50 per cent *of the women using HRT* will get breast cancer.

A similar problem arose when another major research report on breast cancer was leaked to a British national newspaper. The study estimated that women's risk increased by 2.3 per cent for every year of using HRT.[5] The journalist overlooked the fact that this was given as a *percentage* and reported that women on HRT had 2.3 *times* – meaning over double – the risk of developing breast cancer compared to women who weren't on treatment.[6] A frightening idea. It is also easy to come away with the impression that after 10 years of treatment one's risk would *become* 23 per cent, rather than *be up by* about 23 per cent. Again, whatever the increase, it needs to be put into the context of women's risks of breast cancer in the first place.

Assessing women's risks of disease and whether HRT can change these odds is a very technical business. As the rest of this chapter shows, there is considerable debate among doctors and other researchers about the accuracy of risk:benefit information and which type of risk provides the best guide. There is also recognition that because these estimates are based on data from large groups of women, they are limited in their ability to predict what will happen to a given individual. Knowing one's risk of something provides some indication of the future, but that something may never happen.

Finally the risk:benefit equation is not just about numbers. Doctors often despair that women are so concerned about breast cancer when their risk of heart disease is far higher. Doctors' surgeries are full of people with heart disease and heart attack is the main cause of death in countries such as the UK and USA. It tops the medical agenda. Yet the value that women place on avoiding breast cancer is not really surprising given society's attitudes towards cancer or breasts.

What is Heart Disease?

A heart attack occurs when blood flow is disrupted in the arteries that run round the outside of the heart to supply its hard-working muscle. The muscle reacts severely to the lack of oxygen, upsetting the heart's ability to pump blood to the rest of the body. Although the popular image is of immediate death, people tend to survive heart attacks more often than not.

Disruption occurs because fatty deposits have developed in this network of arteries. The process begins when white blood cells and fats collect here and there on the lining of the blood vessels. As the years go by the deposits get bigger, thickening and hardening the elastic walls and narrowing the passage of blood. This is what is meant by 'furring-up of the arteries'. Eventually the deposits may cause irritation, leading to muscle twinges or quite severe spasms in the chest, known as angina. But there may be no signs or symptoms of heart disease until a sudden blockage takes place (heart attack).

Since heart disease doesn't have symptoms in its early stages, researchers have looked for other characteristics that might allow them to make predictions about who was at risk. These characteristics are known as risk factors. Most of them have been studied in men and then applied to women, although it is becoming clear that some risk factors differ for women (see Figure 5.2).

What Has Oestrogen Got to Do with It?

Until recently, heart disease in Westernized countries was seen as a male problem. It is much more likely in men at any age and is their number one cause of death. Hence, it was studied among men. Now there is wider recognition that heart disease also tops the list for women. However, women's pattern of disease is different. For example, American data shows that women develop heart disease 7–10 years later than men and die of it 20 years later.[7] Women are also more likely to develop angina in the first instance, whereas men tend

Figure 5.2 Risk factors for heart disease

If doctors look at a group of people without symptoms and use the following risk factors to predict who will go on to develop heart disease, they will be right 50 per cent of the time.[8]

- Being older
- Belonging to a family with a history of heart disease
- Being a man
- Being diabetic
- Coming from a lower socio-economic group
- Smoking
- Being overweight
- Having high blood pressure*
- Having high blood levels of some types of cholesterol†
- Lacking exercise

Extra risk factors for women:
- Having one's ovaries removed before the natural menopause
- Premature ovarian failure
- By implication, this includes women who lack hormones because of genetic conditions (although women with Turner syndrome can be at extra risk of heart problems for other reasons too, see page 114)

* High blood pressure is a better predictor of heart disease in men than women.
† HDL cholesterol (Figure 5.3) is a better predictor in women.

to have a heart attack. In general, women suffer far fewer premature deaths from what for them remains a disease of later life. Nevertheless, a woman aged 50 has a 46 per cent risk of having heart disease sometime during the rest of her life and a 31 per cent risk of dying from it.[9]

Recognition of the sex differences in heart disease and the delayed pattern in women encouraged the idea that women are protected from the disease by their hormones. This led to the notion that HRT might extend this protection, in spite of an earlier view that taking oestrogen *increased* the risk of heart disease.

This notion of protective HRT gained ground based on the following findings:

1 Studies reported that women's risk of heart disease doubles if their ovaries are removed before the menopause.[10] This extra risk is reduced for those who take oestrogen therapy after surgery.
2 Many studies observed that women who take oestrogen therapy after the natural menopause appear to have a lower risk. This led to the message in leaflets and magazines that 'HRT can halve your risk of heart disease'.
3 Researchers found evidence to suggest that a protective effect was plausible. For example, oestrogen's ability to improve cholesterol levels and dilate blood vessels might explain a reduction in risk.

The extra risk of heart disease among women who lose their hormones at an early age seems fairly clear (although it may not be due simply to lack of hormones[11]). The findings for women after the natural menopause are still being debated because much of the research is problematic or limited in some way.

Take the example of oestrogen and cholesterol levels. Investigators found that oestrogen therapy can improve the levels of certain types of cholesterol in the blood (see Figure 5.3). This sounds very promising because it suggests that oestrogen lowers one of the risk factors and indirectly reduces 'furring-up of the arteries'. The difficulty is that lowering cholesterol levels yields only about 30 per cent of the protective effect. That is, only a third of the observed reduction in risk could possibly be due to HRT's effect on cholesterol levels. Therefore oestrogen and cholesterol cannot be the whole story. However, oestrogen may make *enough* difference in women with high cholesterol levels.

Researchers have also done experiments that show that oestrogen can dilate blood vessels. One can imagine that stretching a stiff,

Figure 5.3 Oestrogen therapy and cholesterol levels

Taking oestrogen increases 'good' cholesterol and decreases 'bad' cholesterol. 'Good' cholesterol may seem like a contradiction in terms, especially after all those early messages that 'too much cholesterol is bad for you'! Scientists have realized since that there are different types of cholesterol.

Briefly cholesterol is used by cells for all sorts of tasks, including the manufacture of hormones (see Chapter 2). The body gets 20 per cent of its cholesterol from food; the liver makes the rest. Cholesterol is ferried in the blood by lipoproteins (fat/protein molecules named after their high density (HDL) or low density (LDL)). HDLs collect cholesterol from the walls of the arteries; LDLs carry it to the fatty deposits.[12] Raised levels of HDL-cholesterol are seen as 'good' because they are associated with less heart disease; high levels of LDL-cholesterol are 'bad'. Oestrogen therapy increases 'good' HDLs and reduces 'bad' LDLs. This could explain some of its apparent benefit in women with this risk factor.

These findings are also behind the preference some doctors have for prescribing HRT as tablets. Oestrogen taken by mouth undergoes the 'first pass' through the liver (see Chapter 4). Usually the 'first pass' gets a bad press because it is associated with certain side-effects. Yet it may account for the beneficial changes described above because the liver produces 80 per cent of the body's cholesterol. Non-oral forms of HRT may have somewhat less effect because they only undergo the 'second pass' through the liver.[13] Researchers are still trying to assess this question. They are also looking at whether the effect is altered by progestogens in combined HRT.

narrowed artery would allow more blood to flow, so perhaps this is another way in which oestrogen reduces the risk of heart disease? Yet no one knows whether the effects seen in experiments can lead to what doctors call 'clinical outcomes',[14] i.e. actual meaningful differences in heart disease among women.

Problems also arise when looking at the work that led to the message that 'HRT can halve your risk of heart disease'. The studies that found that women who take oestrogen HRT have a lower risk of heart disease have been questioned because they looked at women who had already made personal choices about using HRT. The problem is that women who choose HRT may be different in important ways from those who do not – and these differences could bias the results in an unrandomized study. Perhaps the women on HRT had healthier lifestyles (hence their interest in HRT) or were healthier to begin with (since doctors were unlikely to put them on HRT otherwise). This, rather than HRT, could be the reason for their lower risk of heart disease.

The possibility of a 'healthy-user' effect cannot be ignored, but investigators have replied by emphasizing what was done to ensure that comparable women were studied, even though the projects were not randomized trials. Others have tried to calculate how such bias may have affected the results. They argue that the true benefit may be lower, but not low enough to be sneezed at, e.g. a 30-40 per cent reduction in risk.

Some researchers regard the claims for HRT as overstated none the less. For example, several Australian doctors have argued that most women in the menopause have a low risk of heart disease compared to their risks when older. Furthermore, HRT may not have a lasting effect.[15] In this case, trying to reduce women's risks *during the menopause* may not make a great difference to *later* heart disease.[16] To illustrate the point, they estimated that 106–187 women aged 50 would have to be treated with HRT for 10 years to prevent 1 non-fatal heart attack compared to 27–49 women aged 60 treated for the same length of time (they don't give figures for fatal attacks).

It is true that women's risks increase with age, e.g. 1 in 700 has a fatal heart attack by 50 years, 1 in 14 by 75 years.[17] Whether HRT is protective during treatment alone or has a lingering effect is not yet clear. If the benefit does not last, then HRT may be a better bargain when one is older – assuming one gets that far. The difficulty is that older women are also more likely to get breast cancer (see page 95).

The uncertainty about how long women will benefit has led several researchers to comment that the best strategy may be to treat women who have a high risk of heart disease but a low risk of breast cancer until further information becomes available. These women may be women in the natural menopause with several risk factors for heart disease (see Figure 5.2), but no immediate relatives who developed breast cancer before reaching 50 years. Alternatively they may be women who have lacked hormones from an early age. These women have twice the risk of heart disease compared to their friends, but a lower likelihood of breast cancer (see page 95). Here doctors readily advise HRT.

Several studies have looked at a related question: can HRT benefit women with established heart disease (e.g. angina), who are at most risk of a heart attack? Early investigations implied that it could, but the results of a large randomized controlled trial, known as the HERS study, have sent researchers back to the drawing board.[18] This study looked at the effects of combined HRT or placebo over four years in women with an average age of 67. It found that combined HRT did *not* prevent heart attacks in women with established heart disease and caused serious problems more frequently than usual in the first year of treatment (such as thrombosis, which may be more likely in such women, and gall-bladder disease). The researchers concluded that women with established heart disease should not start HRT, but those already beyond one year of treatment could continue. Other large randomized trials are going on now that may provide further answers – in time.

What is Osteoporosis?

Osteoporosis is often described as 'brittle bone' disease. As this name implies, it is a condition in which bones are more likely to crack or break. This comes about because of changes in the microscopic structure of bones such as the spine, hips and wrists.

Bones are designed to be strong but they must also be light, if only

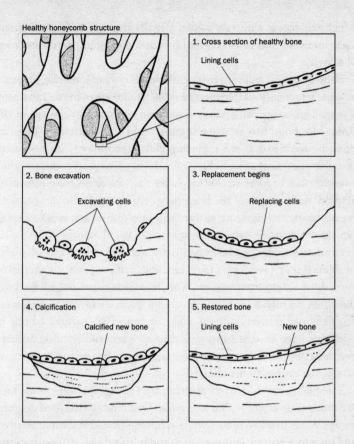

Figure 5.4 Excavating and replacing bone

because they have to be carried around! Certain bones have evolved an internal honeycomb structure for this reason. Like the arches that hold up the vaulted ceiling of a cathedral, this elaborate network of hardened tissue gives bone the capacity to withstand an enormous amount of weight or strain without being too heavy itself. Unlike a ceiling, this architecture is renewed constantly (see Figure 5.4). One type of cell excavates the bone, followed by another type of cell, which replaces it with new tissue. Usually this turnover takes about eight months[19] and bone is built up or lost depending on the balance of activity.

Bone density is built up from childhood onwards, reaching a peak in 25–35-year-olds. After the age of 40, it decreases by 1–2 per cent a year. This could add up to a 30 per cent reduction by the age of 70. This slow bone loss is what scientists call the age-related decline. Bone is lost because the replacing cells (osteoblasts) do not keep up with the excavating cells (osteoclasts). Eventually the internal structure can become so thin in places that the excavating cells may actually remove part of the bony network. The gap remains because the replacing cells have no surface to begin restoration work. This is typical of advanced osteoporosis.

Dramatic as it sounds, bone loss is not a problem as such. The problem is that it is not easy to reverse and, as it progresses, it increases the risk of a 'fragility fracture'. This type of fracture occurs because the bones become less able to withstand ordinary physical pressures. For example, normally one would not expect to fracture a bone if one trips over or when lifting a child or groceries. If osteoporosis becomes very severe, women can crack bones by getting in and out of a car or rising from a chair.

The places most likely to fracture because of excessive bone loss are the spinal vertebrae, hip and wrist. One tends to think of doctors setting bones to allow them to repair, but hip fractures are inaccessible and therefore require major surgery and hospital care. Complications are frequent and will be fatal for 20 per cent of patients. Survivors face a slow recovery and the challenge of regaining their mobility. According to one estimate, only 50 per cent of women recover enough to live independently.[20] Spinal fractures are less dangerous and demand less hospital care, but they can be very debilitating. Back pain is common and curvature of the spine can cause breathing and digestive problems as the upper body presses forward. Women may be mobile but everyday tasks can become difficult.

Whether bone loss becomes a problem that places one at risk depends on several things, not least how much bone one has to start with. People who build up more bone by their thirties have less risk of later fracture. This can depend on one's genetic background. For example, men build up more bone than women and black women build up more bone than Asian, Chinese or white women. Which isn't to say that men and black women can't get osteoporosis, but it is less likely. A family inheritance of smaller frames or a history of osteoporosis can also play a part.

Cultural factors such as diet and weight-bearing exercise also affect how much bone is deposited. For example, the body uses dietary calcium to build bones and regular (i.e. three times a week) weight-bearing exercise appears to stimulate bone-replacing cells. Indeed, stress and strain appear to be vital for bone formation. This seems rather clever; after all, few road bridges get stronger when carrying more cars! Though one can see why lack of exercise doesn't help – and why astronauts suffer bone loss if they remain weightless for too long.

The build-up of bone is also altered by the production of sex hormones in puberty. Young women who lack hormones or lose them early are likely to reach a low peak bone mass by their late thirties and have a high risk of developing osteoporosis and later fractures (unless they receive long-term HRT). A less prolonged lack of periods, perhaps due to athlete training or anorexia, can also interrupt the build-up of peak bone mass.

The age-related decline is a greater potential problem for women than men because they build up less bone to begin with and tend to live longer. Also, the decline for women has a dip in it after the natural menopause. However, the effects of the natural menopause and longevity need to be kept in perspective. For example, data on fracture rates in different countries suggest that genetic differences and cultural lifestyles are more important than whether one is a woman or a man.[21] Similarly researchers regard poorer quality bone, not longer lives, as the reason behind the threefold increase in the incidence of fractures among women over the last 30 years in Europe (the rise is even greater for men).

Of course, the risk of fractures is not just about better bones or bone loss. Hip fractures are also about why older people fall. This may be due to the effects of ageing such as poorer eyesight, less fitness and slower reaction times.[22] Yet women seem to fall more often than men. The use of tranquillizers or sedatives, lack of safety in the home/ residential home and women's footwear may be important factors.

Forecasting Fractures

Doctors can use risk factors to judge whether someone is likely to suffer a later fracture, but they also try to assess this more directly by measuring bone loss. Many leaflets on osteoporosis have a graphic picture showing that the internal structure of bone has become thread-bare and developed gaps. Doctors cannot take such a picture in a living person. Instead they diagnose osteoporosis by measuring bone mineral density (BMD). A bone loses density as it thins, so density is a guide to its strength.

Bone mineral density results are analysed and recorded in terms of either standard deviations or percentages of an average value. In other words, osteoporosis is defined using statistics rather than symptoms (see Figure 5.5). This sounds rather off-putting – even if one is curious about the meaning of one's bone scan results! Yet if curiosity prevails, one only needs to be equipped with a bit of information about averages and standard deviations. It is enough to know that the average is a way of judging what is typical in a group, e.g. the average height in a class of children. The standard deviation (SD) is calculated to gauge how unusual something is compared to what is typical, e.g. the spread of heights compared to the average height in class.

It may help to stay with the example of height for a moment to see how statistical comparisons can be useful. For example, a child's growth can be compared with what is typical using national statistics on height. A child who has not grown as much as expected may need further investigation, which could diagnose a condition such as Turner syndrome. Of course, children can be shorter than average and *not* have a health problem. That is, height measurements can offer useful warnings rather than cast-iron predictions.

Figure 5.5 How osteoporosis is defined

1993 Consensus conference

'Disease characterized by low bone mass and micro-architectural deterioration of bone tissue leading to enhanced bone fragility and consequent increase in fracture risk.'

1994 World Health Organisation

Average bone mass:	within 1 SD of average for young adults (T score)
Low bone mass (osteopenia):	between −1 and −2 SDs below this average
Osteoporosis:	between −2 and −2.5 SDs below this average
Severe osteoporosis:	at least −2.5 SDs, with fragility fractures

For each reduction of 1 standard deviation (SD), the risk of fracture doubles.[23]

Bone-density measurements can also provide useful warnings. Much as described for height, someone's bone density can be compared with what is typical. In this case, several comparisons can be made to help decide whether a person has osteoporosis and predict their risk of future fractures. The first is with young adults of the same sex (T score, see Figure 5.5). Young adults have peak bone mass, so this means that someone's bone density is being compared with typical peak bone mass. Their result can also be compared with what is typical for others of the same age and sex (Z score).

Using the T scores shown in Figure 5.5, one can see that osteoporosis is defined as bone density more than 2 SDs below average. The risk of fracture doubles with each SD, so women with osteoporosis have four times the average risk of a later fracture. However, this diagnosis and forecast needs to be interpreted with care. For example, it has been estimated that of the 20 per cent with the lowest bone density, only a quarter will have a later fracture.[24] Equally two-thirds of those who have a fracture will be patients previously judged *not* at risk.

Having a Bone Scan

Bone density can be measured by passing radiation or ultrasound through bone tissue, rather as one might check the density of a sheet of paper against the light. Standard X-rays show bone loss only when it is greater than 30 per cent, so more sensitive DXA scanners were developed. These machines use about a tenth of the radiation of a chest X-ray. QCT scanners (or CAT scanners) can also be adapted to measure bone density, although they use more radiation.

Women referred to a hospital for a DXA bone scan will find the experience straightforward. One is advised to wear clothes without metal buttons, studs or underwiring (zips are OK), and then invited to rest on a special couch for 10–20 minutes while a mechanical arm takes the measurements. There is no alarming equipment, no tunnel and no need for the radiographer to retreat.

However, DXA machines are expensive and the scans themselves don't come cheap since they are slow and require skilled staff. The search is on for convenient tests that could become more widely available. For example, a smaller, potentially portable machine has been developed that does a quick heel check. Heel checks can also be done more frequently as they use ultrasound rather than radiation. Researchers are still trying to assess whether the results provide reliable predictions about the risk of fractures.

There are several other problems with the measurement of bone density. Firstly, the results of DXA, QCT and heel scans cannot be compared because they take readings in different ways. Secondly, scans should be repeated on the same machine if possible (not just the same type), otherwise variations in the results may have more to do with switching machines than personal changes in bone density. Different manufacturers use different population data to make the statistical comparisons and even machines of the same type have varying error rates.

Then there is the question of which bone(s) to measure. In short, bones vary in the way they are affected by bone loss. Some sites are better 'oracles' when it comes to predicting the risk of future fractures or monitoring someone's response to treatment. For example, current treatments do not affect bone turnover in the heel, so heel measurements are rather irrelevant in this case. Changes in bone turnover show up most readily in the spine.

DXA machines usually measure the hip and spine, the two most common sites for future fractures. Spine measurements tend to be more accurate[25] and can also provide a better prediction of who is at risk. However, in general, if one wants to predict the chances of a hip fracture, then one is better off looking at a *hip* result and likewise for the spine. This is true unless the bone has already suffered a fracture, in which case it can give a misleading measurement, particularly in the spine. In older women, where this is more likely, doctors can concentrate on hip measurements.

Given some of the drawbacks of bone scans, the possibility of measuring relevant substances in the blood or urine is being investigated. Some test-kits have even come on to the market, although there are little data as yet about their ability to make meaningful forecasts of the risk of later fractures.

Who Should Be Scanned?

Osteoporosis receives a lot of publicity and so women are beginning to ask themselves whether they should be having bone scans after the menopause. This is understandable, since learning about a graphic problem such as 'brittle bones' can provoke anxiety. Magazine articles and radio phone-ins can suggest that all one has to do is beat a path to the doctor and ask for a bone scan. The message is that if women are concerned, they should be screened. This may relieve women's anxiety, but is it a good way of solving the problem of osteoporosis? As this section explains, the answer is 'no'.

Figure 5.6 Who is eligible for screening using DXA bone scans?

UK Department of Health guidelines[26] recommend that doctors refer only groups at high risk of osteoporosis for screening with DXA bone scans. Among women these broadly include:

- women who have had a surgical, medical or natural menopause before the age of 45
- women who have had a hysterectomy leaving one or both ovaries before the age of 45
- women who have missed their periods for six months or more (for reasons other than pregnancy)
- women who lack hormones due to primary hypogonadism (e.g. Turner syndrome)
- post-menopausal women with other risk factors for osteoporosis
- women who have had previous fragility fractures

There are several reasons for not scanning every woman – or even every woman who wants this test. Some reasons are to do with bone scans and some are to do with HRT. As the previous sections have shown, bone scans are limited in their ability to make predictions about who is at risk and therefore who would benefit from treatment. If they were used to screen everyone, many predictions would be wrong (see pages 89–90). Some people would be worried and treated unnecessarily; others would be missed having been given the all-clear. In short, a better test is needed before screening everyone becomes ethical. However, bone scans provide more reliable predictions when they are done in high-risk groups (see Figure 5.6). These groups have been chosen as eligible for five-yearly NHS bone scans according to UK Department of Health guidelines.

Yet, it can be argued, even this screening may be unnecessary, given the merits of HRT. Women gain from treatment whatever their bone density, so why bother with a scan? If the result adds up to osteoporosis, HRT will be advised for this reason; if not, HRT will be recommended for its other benefits. Why not just prescribe HRT in the first place? This view explains the lack of enthusiasm that can greet women who arrive in the surgery insisting on a bone scan, especially if they rule out HRT in the same breath.

HRT and Osteoporosis

Lack of sex hormones during the age-related decline increases the number of excavating cells, tipping the balance even further towards bone loss. This suggests that boosting the replacing cells would restore equilibrium, but it has not been easy to find a drug to persuade the body to add bone directly. Most treatments prevent bone loss by slowing down the excavators.

Oestrogen therapy prevents osteoporosis by reducing bone loss. However, researchers are not sure how it does this. Few oestrogen receptors have been found in the excavating cells.[27] Still, these receptors are very attractive to oestrogen, so perhaps it doesn't matter that they are uncommon. Alternatively oestrogen therapy may work indirectly by influencing substances that affect bone loss in turn. In any case, women must be on a sufficient dose of oestrogen to prevent osteoporosis (see Figure 10.1, page 214). Some progestogens may add to the effect of oestrogen.

When women start HRT, their bone density rises about 5–7 per cent in the first year or so and then stays the same for the next few years.[28] Much longer-term effects haven't been studied in detail, but doctors assume that 'bone-sparing' continues during treatment. Ongoing trials will provide further answers, but current assessments are that HRT reduces the risk of a hip fracture by about 30 per cent and a spinal fracture by about 50 per cent.[29] An estimated five years' treatment is required to show a benefit in terms of hip fractures.[30] Ten years' treatment is calculated to prevent a 10–15 per cent drop in bone density which would otherwise be equivalent to a doubling of the fracture risk (i.e. one standard deviation, see Figure 5.5).[31]

The difficulty is that bone loss starts again when women stop HRT. This loss appears to carry on in the same way as before treatment, although some studies suggest that it may be faster. As a result, women could live long enough after treatment to develop low bone density that places them at risk. Indeed, it appears that 10 years after stopping HRT women can end up with the same bone density and risk of later fractures as women who didn't bother.[32]

This poses questions. If women are at most risk of fractures 25 years after the natural menopause, when should they take HRT and for how long? Two Australian doctors calculated that 488–1428 women aged 50 would have to take HRT for 10 years to prevent 1 hip fracture compared to 160–458 women aged 60.[33] Nevertheless, doctors are reluctant to wait to treat their patients because this means resigning them wittingly to a 15–25 per cent loss in bone density in the intervening time.[34] It is apparent that women who lack hormones from an early age need to take HRT until the age of 50 and probably beyond to prevent bone loss. Women in the natural menopause who are at high risk of osteoporosis for other reasons may also benefit from HRT at this stage. The equations for women without menopausal symptoms or a high risk of osteoporosis are less clear.

HRT is regarded as the 'gold standard' for osteoporosis, but other treatments exist, notably the biphosphonates such as Fosamax (alendronate) and Didronel (etidronate). Biphosphonates reduce excavation and thus prevent bone loss. Fosamax can be awkward to take (see Kate, Chapter 1). The best length of treatment is not yet clear, but it may be up to seven years.[35]

What is Breast Cancer?

Cancer develops when cell division goes awry. Most body cells are replaced many times during someone's lifetime. The new cells are exact replicas and produced only when needed. However, problems can arise if they become altered genetically during division. In this case, they may not grow according to plan and cancer can form.

Cancer is more likely as people get older, partly because they have been through more cell replacement in which mistakes may have occurred. For example, the risk of dying from breast cancer before the age of 25 is 1 in 200,000. This increases to 1 in 200 by age 50 and 1 in 30 by age 75.[36] Indeed, for most women, *age* is by far the most important risk factor for breast cancer. However, women can have an extra risk of the disease if an immediate relative had breast cancer before the age of 50. A few women have an exceptional risk because they have the BRCA1 gene.

Women's risk of breast cancer is also related to when they reach the menopause. For example, women who reach the menopause before they turn 45 have half the risk of breast cancer compared to women who have a late menopause (after the age of 55). Their risk appears to be related to the length of time they are exposed to their own oestrogen. This could be because oestrogen increases cell division in the breast.[37] When there is more cell division, an error is slightly more likely to occur and if it does, it will grow into a tumour more quickly (although this may still take 10–15 years). This suggests that oestrogen does not *cause* the genetic alterations that lead to cancer cells, but could alter the chances of them occurring.

HRT and Breast Cancer

Breast cancer is the risk associated with taking HRT that worries women. Since oestrogen is associated with breast cancer, this is not an unreasonable fear. Studies on the subject have produced conflicting results, hence a lot of debate. Finally work was published that pooled and re-analysed data from many different studies,[38] and concluded that women aged 50–70 who use HRT do have a slight additional risk of developing breast cancer. The extra risk varies according to the length of treatment and wears off within five years of stopping HRT (see Figure 5.7). Progestogens do not appear to counter the effects of oestrogen here, unlike their ability to reduce the extra risk of endometrial cancer.

Figure 5.7 Predicted effect of HRT on breast cancer in women aged 50–70*

The existing risk

In those not using HRT, about 45 in every 1000 women aged 50 will have breast cancer diagnosed over the next 20 years.

The additional risk

In those using HRT
- for five years, the figure above rises by 2 women to 47 in every 1000 women
- for ten years, it rises by 6 women to 51 in every 1000 women
- for fifteen years, it rises by 12 women to 57 in every 1000 women who will have breast cancer diagnosed over the next 20 years.

  After stopping HRT it takes about five years for women's chances to return to their background risk. Several randomized trials are going on which may provide further guidance.

(Source: British National Formulary, March 1998)

*Women on HRT from an early age, see page 95.

The information in Figure 5.7 makes alarming reading for women who have been on HRT from an early age unless it is put into context (which no one troubled to do when it was leaked to the newspapers). As described above, all younger women have a lower risk of breast cancer because of their age. Younger women who lack hormones or lose them early (see Chapters 6–8) appear to have an even *lower* risk, having had no or less exposure to their own oestrogen. Therefore doctors believe that HRT does no more than return a younger woman's risk to roughly what it would have been had she not lost her hormones.

She will only begin to have any extra risk of breast cancer when she is 50 years old and then only in the same way as other women on HRT after the menopause. This conclusion is an educated guess by doctors since it has not been the subject of research, partly because of the difficulty involved in finding large numbers of women in this position and following them over time. Doctors are clear that women who lack hormones from an early age need HRT since they have extra risks of osteoporosis and heart disease compared to women who have a natural menopause.

Figure 5.7 suggests that women aged 50–70 can use HRT for several years without adding too much to their existing risk of breast cancer. However, their other benefits will be limited unless they use HRT for longer. Although it may not be a consolation, women who *do* develop breast cancer while on HRT appear to be more likely to survive the disease. There could be several reasons for this finding. Some researchers think that the type of breast cancer seen in women on HRT is less likely to spread. Others have argued that better survival could be an *indirect* result of being on HRT. For example, doctors may spot a potential problem if they are monitoring patients on HRT. Women may pick up cancer earlier because being on HRT makes them more vigilant about any changes in their breasts.

Breast Screening

Current UK Department of Health guidance is that there is no need to regard women on HRT as a special case when it comes to screening for breast cancer. At present the National Breast Screening Programme invites women aged 50–64 for a mammogram every three years. The reasons for inviting this age group are not obvious and easily cause misunderstanding. Of course, any woman who is worried about changes in her breasts, such as an unfamiliar lump, can gain access to a specialist through her GP.

As discussed earlier, age is the best guide to one's risk of developing breast cancer. Research has shown that screening women aged 50–64 provides more overall benefit, as a result of catching and treating cancer earlier, than the harm done either by worrying women in the first place or by conducting further investigations that will prove unnecessary in some cases. Women over 65 years can request regular screening, even though they are not invited routinely.

The position for women under 50 is rather different. They are not invited by the national screening programme because the chances of finding breast cancer in younger women are too low to warrant mass screening (although women with a strong family history may be referred in some cases). Even if such a programme was funded, it would run into the difficulties of doing mammograms in pre-menopausal women.

One of the problems is that breast tissue changes during the menopause. Before the menopause the many tiny ducts throughout the breasts respond to hormonal fluctuations during the menstrual cycle. After the menopause, these ducts fade and the tissue becomes much less dense. The change can be seen on a mammogram: dense tissue looks quite cloudy; later the picture clears. Since cloudy mammograms are harder to interpret, more mistaken results would come about in a screening programme for pre-menopausal women. This is one of the reasons why a screening programme for younger women is regarded as unjustified.

Perhaps not surprisingly women on HRT can have cloudy mammograms.[39] This finding has led to some controversy about whether women should have a mammogram before starting HRT, to allow radiographers to compare later pictures. In the USA women are given HRT only after a normal mammogram.[40] In the UK many health professionals involved with breast screening agree with this approach, although it is not advocated in present guidance from the Department of Health's Advisory Committee on Breast Cancer Screening.[41]

6

INTERRUPTED SEXUAL DEVELOPMENT

'I cry over the fact that at a time of life when all my friends got their periods, I instead got a pill. I didn't want "womanhood from a bottle". I desperately wanted to cross the threshold into womanhood in the same way as my friends did – by having a menstrual cycle.'

SHERRI GROVEMAN

Women may turn to this chapter in disbelief. For some, it will be the first time they have found a health book that recognizes the problems they face. Others may arrive at this page out of curiosity. A well-meaning curiosity, but one that several women in this chapter learnt to avoid or fear because their condition has been shrouded in secrecy by society, doctors and others. Such secrecy has often imposed an appalling burden, leading to years of silent confusion and painful isolation. It has also meant that other people have not had a chance to recognize that these conditions exist or understand how women can feel.

This chapter describes how a baby girl grows in her mother's womb and what happens if her sexual development is interrupted at this stage. Different interruptions lead to different medical conditions. For example, she may be born without ovaries, with 'streak' ovaries or with testes. However, most of the women here share the problem of missing hormones; some need HRT from adolescence onwards. Those *with* ovaries, but without a womb or vagina, may be at risk of a premature menopause (see Mary, below).

However, a medical explanation isn't everything. Helpful though it is to understand what happens during sexual development, this chapter is also about what it *means* to be a woman with one of these conditions. Here, women speak for themselves.

Becoming a Girl

When an egg meets a sperm, they fuse into the first cell of a new human being. This cell unites the chromosomes they bring from each parent. Chromosomes contain genetic instructions, including those that guide early development.

Usually the first cell has 46 chromosomes, including a pair of sex chromosomes. There are two kinds of sex chromosome: an X or the smaller Y chromosome (see Figure 6.1). Eggs carry an X chromosome. Sperm carry an X *or* a Y.

If an egg meets an X-carrying sperm, the embryo will be XX and can grow into a girl or an intersex baby. If it meets a Y-carrying sperm, it will be XY and can grow into a boy, a girl or an intersex baby. In other words, the sperm cell influences the genetic sex of the baby – a fact that might have enlightened King Henry VIII, who allegedly blamed his *wives* for producing daughters before a male heir.

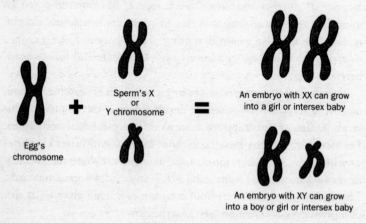

Egg's chromosome

+

Sperm's X or Y chromosome

=

An embryo with XX can grow into a girl or intersex baby

An embryo with XY can grow into a boy or girl or intersex baby

Figure 6.1 There are two types of sex chromosome

Soon after fertilization, the first cell divides in two. Each cell divides again and again: four, eight, 16 cells and so on. Every cell gets a copy of all the chromosomes. As the ball of cells multiplies, it moves down the Fallopian tube to the womb, where it implants itself in the lining and continues to grow. Slowly the cells become guided by different parts of their copy of the genetic instructions. Their appearance begins to vary. Groups start to gather and move to new positions. As they change and rearrange themselves into early structures, the embryo begins to take shape.

Several cell clusters are needed for future sex organs (see Figure 6.2). First to appear is a pair of primitive 'male' ducts, one on either side of the embryo near the tail. Two long bundles emerge to mark nearby sites for ovaries or testes (A). Then the 'male' ducts attach their lower ends to another developing cluster, the future genitals. The next stage seems bizarre: a group of future egg/sperm cells moves from the yolk sac across the embryo to settle on the two long bundles, which will house them as ovaries or testes eventually (see B and B side view).

About a week later, a pair of primitive 'female' ducts begin to follow the 'male' ducts down to the genital cluster. Half-way there, the 'female' ducts grow towards each other. Once alongside, they complete the journey to the genital cluster where they form a solid tip anchored between the 'male' ducts (C). By the time everything is in place, the embryo is seven weeks old.

At this stage most of the structures described are neutral. That is, the future egg/sperm, ovaries/testes and genitals are yet to become male, female or, more occasionally, intersex. In contrast, the primitive ducts appear in male *and* female versions in the embryo. This means that one duct system must be developed and the other dismantled before birth. These changes are controlled initially by the sex chromosomes and, later, by hormones. Genetic instructions direct the cells due to become eggs or sperm and hence stored as ovaries or testes. If the instruction is for testes and testes grow accordingly, they make hormones for male development of the ducts and genitals.

Sexual development begins after the seventh week of life. If the genetic code is XX, then eggs and ovaries form. Without testes and male hormones, the 'male' duct system dissolves away (see Figure 6.2). The upper 'female' ducts become two Fallopian tubes. In the middle, where the ducts run alongside, they fuse, thicken and hollow into a uterus above the solid tip and the genital cluster. The genital cluster elongates away from this anchored tip to form a solid vagina. By the fifth month the vagina has also hollowed out, leaving the cervix at the top of the vagina and hymen at its entrance. As Figure 6.3 shows, the cervix and upper vagina come from the solid tip of the 'female' duct system, whereas the lower vagina comes from the genital cluster. Meanwhile, the genitals have grown into the inner and outer lips of the vulva and the clitoris.

It is remarkable to think that the genital cell cluster could have grown into a penis, instead of a clitoris, and sealed its folds of skin into a scrotum to hold testes (which descend from the abdomen to form testicles), instead of opening them further into the double lips of the vulva (see Figure 6.4). However, male development requires a Y chromosome to instruct the growth of testes. Then the testes must produce male hormones to stimulate the 'male' duct system, erase the 'female' version and convert the genitals. Without these chemical signals, female organs develop. In other words, embryos always become female, irrespective of their genetic sex, unless they receive male hormonal messages. Sometimes this is called the Eve principle because the fundamental form for the human body is female.

The reasons for the Eve principle are unclear. Some authors suggest that female development is stimulated by oestrogens circulating in the mother's body and placenta (perhaps as well as from the embryo's ovaries).[1] In this case, one can see why male hormones are needed to ensure the baby is male! Whatever the reason, the Eve principle and the way sex organs grow from different cell clusters (in response to genetic and/or hormonal instructions) help to explain why such organs can occur in intersex combinations or be partially missing.

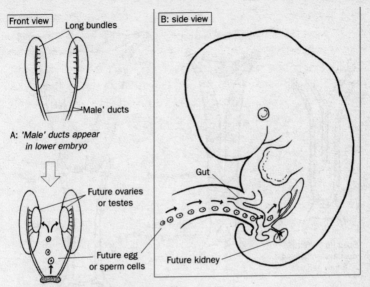

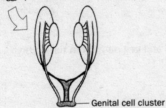

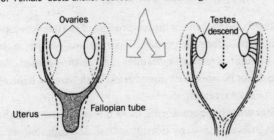

Figure 6.2 Growth of cell clusters for future sex organs

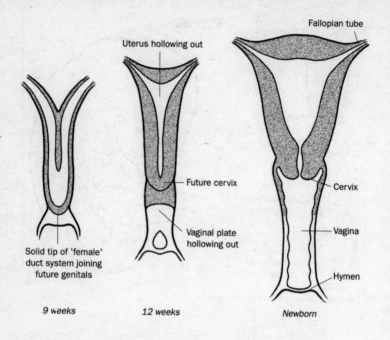

Figure 6.3 The way the uterus and vagina grow in the embryo

Interrupted Development

Perhaps it isn't surprising that the complex process of sexual development can skip a step. Either the genetic instructions or the male hormonal messages that direct later changes may be interrupted. As a result, a baby girl can be born without ovaries, with 'streak' ovaries or with testes instead of ovaries.

Before looking at what happens during these interruptions, it might be helpful to imagine all the steps during sexual development as a long line of dominoes standing upright next to each other. Pushing over the first domino may cause each domino to fall, in order, until the very last. Except that life isn't like that. Often the dominoes fall

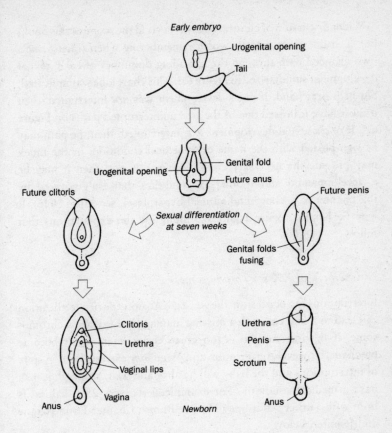

Figure 6.4 Male and female genitals grow from the same early structure

until an interruption stops the cascade or some of the dominoes start falling in unexpected ways. Whether these other patterns are acceptable can depend on whether the emphasis is on reaching the last domino. For example, Western society tends to see sexual development as ending with two last dominoes, male and female, even though the dominoes have always fallen – and are still falling – into other patterns. This is a *value* judgement that ignores biological reality.

Wider discussion of cultural issues is beyond the scope of this book, but such questions may be worth remembering when tracing one's own chanced path through the cascading dominoes of early sexual development summarized in Figure 6.5. This chart looks complicated, but help is at hand. If one's development was *not* interrupted, then it must have followed one of the two uninterrupted paths on Figure 6.5. If one's sexual development *was* interrupted, then the path may be sign-posted with the name of a medical condition, or the Index may provide the necessary cross-reference. If not, then it may be a developmental and/or intersex condition that isn't covered by this chapter (e.g. congenital adrenal hyperplasia, see More Help). It may be helpful to use Figure 6.5 alongside the explanations that follow.

Girls with X or XX sex chromosomes

Interruptions can occur from the word go. An upset during fertilization can lead to a first cell with a missing, damaged or extra sex chromosome. If the interruption is too great, the woman won't become pregnant. However, fertilization and pregnancy can go ahead in spite of interruptions and the baby will be alive and well, although it may have a medical condition. For example, 1 in every 2500 babies[2] is born with Turner syndrome (TS) (see Bungy, Chapter 1 and Joanne and Jennifer, below).

'Syndrome' is the word for a pattern of things that happen together and Turner syndrome is named after the man who published a modern description of it. Women with TS share a pattern of signs: usually they are born without functioning ovaries and grow to be shorter than average (especially without growth hormone treatment). However, they can have other associated problems (see More Help).

'Classic' or 'complete' Turner syndrome occurs when an interruption during fertilization causes one of the sex chromosomes to 'drop off' as the egg and sperm cell merge (see Figure 6.5). The first cell of the new baby is left with an X – rather than XX or XY. Usually the X is from the mother's egg having lost the father's X or Y chromosome,

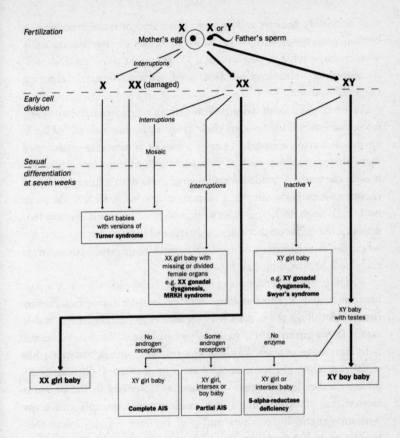

Figure 6.5 Some of the cascading dominoes of early sexual development

but in a third of cases[3] the remaining X comes from an X-carrying sperm. Either way, the baby's genetic sex is written as 45,X (or 45,X0) to show that her body cells have 45 (rather than 46) chromosomes and one X in the sex chromosome 'pair'.

Sometimes the first cell *does* have a second sex chromosome, but it has been damaged before or during fertilization. The chromosome may be visibly broken and/or have lost some of its instructions. A broken chromosome is more likely to be an X, but occasionally women have what is known as a 'Y fragment', i.e. a piece of Y chromosome. This can be associated with a tumour, requiring surgery.[4]

About 50 per cent of women with Turner syndrome have a missing sex chromosome in *some* of their body cells, but not all.[5] This is known as having a *mosaic*. Usually a mosaic is a picture made up of many different pieces, such as coloured tiles or beads. Here, 'mosaic' means the body is made of millions of cells with slightly different chromosomes. For example, a woman who is 45,X/46,XX has some body cells with 45,X and others with 46,XX. It is as if she has two genetic colours throughout her body instead of one. A mosaic occurs when the interruption occurs slightly later than fertilization, when early cells are dividing (see Figure 6.5).

Whatever the interruption at this stage, baby girls who lack a pair of undamaged X chromosomes will be born without functioning ovaries. Although the ovaries may fill with eggs (see Figure 6.2, B side view), they tend to die off early. This can have different effects: the baby may have ovaries that lack egg follicles, 'streak' ovaries (thin streaks of white fibrous tissue), or no sign of ovaries. Girls with TS do have other female organs because, as described in the previous section, the 'female' duct system and external genitals can grow without genetic instructions and will become female unless they receive male hormonal messages to the contrary. The 'male' duct system dissolves away in the absence of a Y chromosome (although a Y fragment may lead to a remaining tumour).

Sometimes, girls are born without ovaries or with 'streak' ovaries even though later genetic tests show they have a pair of undamaged X chromosomes. This suggests growth was interrupted for some other reason (see Figure 6.5). This can be known as XX gonadal dysgenesis.[6] Just as apples and oranges can be called fruit, ovaries and testes can be called *gonads* (after the Greek *gonos* for 'seed'). 'Dysgenesis' means the gonads haven't 'become' (Greek *gen*), although no one really knows why not.

Development of the ovaries is not the only stage that can be interrupted. Looking back at the way the 'female' duct system grows, it becomes easier to see how a semi-divided or double uterus can occur if the ducts don't merge or hollow out (see Figure 6.6). An estimated 1 in every 1500 women has a uterus that shows some variation,[7] although many cases may remain undiagnosed because usually they don't cause problems. An altered uterine shape can cause repeated miscarriage and, very occasionally, surgery is needed to allow menstruation.

Growth of the genital cell cluster can also be interrupted. For example, a double cervix or double vagina can occur if the vagina

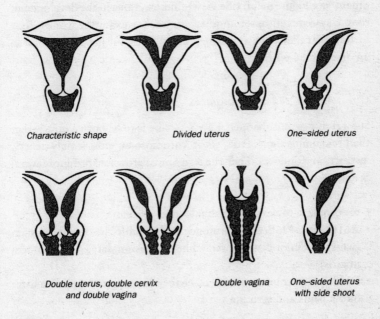

Characteristic shape   *Divided uterus*   *One–sided uterus*

Double uterus, double cervix   *Double vagina*   *One–sided uterus*
and double vagina   *with side shoot*

Figure 6.6 The uterus and vagina can vary in shape if their growth is interrupted

doesn't hollow out as expected (see Figure 6.6). Sometimes a slightly bulging membrane simply covers the vaginal opening, situated above the hymen. Girls born without vaginal depth may or may not have a partially formed uterus. Some women born without vaginas have MRKH or Mayer-Rokitansky-Kuster-Hauser syndrome (see Mary, below), a condition named to honour several medical scientists, which gives patients rather a tongue-twister.[8] These women have XX chromosomes and therefore ovaries, but *may* be at risk of an early menopause.[9]

Women may find that doctors wish to X-ray their kidneys when trying to diagnose these conditions. This can seem odd until one realizes that the kidneys and bladder develop alongside the early sex organs (see Figure 6.2, B side view). Interruptions in the development of one system can upset another and so, for example, women may be told that they have a missing kidney or that it has been found in an unexpected position.

Girls with XY sex chromosomes

Several things must happen if an XY baby is to be born a boy, rather than remaining a girl. First, the Y chromosome must supply genetic instructions for testes. Then the testes must grow and produce several hormones:

- testosterone to develop the 'male' duct system
- AMH (anti-Müllerian hormone) to dismantle the 'female' system (which does not dissolve away like the unstimulated 'male' system in girls)
- DHT (dihydrotestosterone) to change the external genital cluster into a penis and scrotum

Several kinds of interruption can occur during this process which mean that the embryo remains female. For example, occasionally the Y chromosome doesn't become active enough (see Figure 6.5). The testes may begin to grow but then shrink. This may be because the short arm of the Y is damaged and unable to produce the supposed testes-determining factor (TDF).[10] Early lack of growth leads to the birth of a girl with XY gonadal dysgenesis (for XX equivalent, see page 108) or Swyer's syndrome.[11] These girls are born without ovaries, which need XX, and without testes, which need TDF. Sometimes girls have 'streaks' of tissue (see Juanita, below). Since they do not have testes, they do not produce AMH to dismantle their 'female' duct system. In this case, given the Eve principle, the 'female' duct system goes ahead and develops into Fallopian tubes, a uterus and upper vagina. The genital cluster forms the lower vagina, clitoris and vulva.

A different interruption occurs when the Y chromosome does become active and the embryo's testes do grow, but are missing an enzyme (5-alpha-reductase deficiency). This means her testes can make some, but not all, of the hormones needed for male development, i.e. AMH and testosterone, but not the related hormone DHT. Without DHT, her genitals will become female or intersex. However, unlike the baby above, she has AMH, and this hormone dismantles her 'female' duct system. As a result, she loses the chance of having Fallopian tubes, a womb and upper vagina.

Sometimes, an embryo's testes produce all the necessary enzymes and hormones for male development, but the testosterone and DHT messages cannot be *read* by the 'male' duct system or genitals (see Rosemary, Chapter 1, and Sherri and Rosie, below). This may be because there are no receptors for the androgen hormones or such receptors aren't working (androgen insensitivity syndrome (AIS), previously called testicular feminization (TF), among other things). Either way, the androgen 'keys' cannot 'unlock' development (see Chapter 2). Without stimulation, the 'male' ducts dissolve away. However, like the baby above, her testes will produce AMH. This hormone dismantles most or all of her 'female' duct system so that she will be born without Fallopian tubes, a womb or upper vagina.

Girls with 'complete' AIS (CAIS) have a clitoris, vulva and lower vagina (which women with CAIS say can be very short or almost full-length). 'Partial' AIS (PAIS) means there are *some* active androgen receptors (see Figure 6.5) and therefore some tissues may have responded to the male hormones. This is why girls and women with 'partial' AIS can have genitals that vary in shape. For example, the vaginal lips may be partially fused and the clitoris may be enlarged. Some babies with PAIS appear intersex or male. Detailed discussion of PAIS is outside the scope of this book (see More Help).

Girls and women with AIS and related conditions have received very hurtful newspaper headlines such as 'The boy sentenced to live inside a schoolgirl's body'.[12] Women with AIS say that they *can* feel trapped, but not because of the idea that they are somehow males trying to get out. Instead, they describe feeling trapped by secrecy and silence, to say nothing of society's confused attitudes towards sexual difference, gender and sexuality. Some also feel trapped by not having full-length vaginas and the comparative lack of medical research in this area. Furthermore, as they point out, the success of genital surgery has often been defined in terms of 'cosmetic normality and penetrative sex' rather than maintaining the ability to orgasm.[13]

(Women with TS complain about equally hurtful and unoriginal publicity ('Woman trapped in child's body').[14] Again, they feel that this says more about a society that values women who are 'fertile, tall, slim and blonde'[15] than it does about the experience of having Turner syndrome.)

Becoming a Woman

Biologically there are two stages of sexual development: becoming a baby girl and becoming a woman. As described above, the first stage is controlled by one's sex chromosomes and then various hormones within the embryo. The second stage, puberty, is controlled by hormones alone and depends on what happened during the first stage.

A girl begins puberty during late childhood when her hypothalamus, a gland just below the brain, produces a hormone called GnRH. At first, she releases GnRH every so often at night. Slowly her pulses of hormone become more frequent, appearing during the day as well.

Eventually the pulses become strong enough to prompt the pituitary to produce pulses of another hormone, FSH. The ovaries respond to FSH by producing low levels of oestrogen, which stimulate breast development, enlarge the womb and thicken its lining. As time goes on, her fat distribution changes as her breasts and hips round out and she develops soft padding over her pubic bone. The lips of her vulva elongate and the lining of her vagina becomes capable of producing extra lubrication during sexual excitement. On average, her first period appears between the ages of 11 and 15. This tends to be after the growth of her pubic hair, but before the appearance of under-arm hair.

About 5 per cent of girls with Turner syndrome have ovaries and produce enough oestrogen for puberty to take place (see Joanne, below); a few menstruate for a while.[16] However, most girls with TS need hormone replacement from their early teenage years to experience these changes. This should be undertaken under the guidance of a specialist and preferably in consultation with the girl and her family.[17]

Usually a girl is given a low dose of oestrogen that is increased over a year or two to stimulate breast development and build up the lining of her womb. Some blood spotting may occur before a progestogen is added for 12 days each month; if not, this second hormone will start her periods. Doctors call these 'withdrawal bleeds' because bleeding is produced by withdrawing progestogen each month. At this stage, she may be prescribed a 'low-dose' contraceptive pill or, more rarely, a reduced dose of HRT. When she is older, she may be given a higher-dose Pill or a combined form of HRT.

The idea of using the contraceptive pill may be confusing until one thinks about the way it works. The Pill is designed to control the menstrual cycle so that a woman doesn't ovulate but continues to have regular 'periods'. Put another way, it prompts a woman's body to have regular withdrawal bleeds even though she is not ovulating, and so it can be used to generate a menstrual cycle in women without functioning ovaries. HRT can also be used to do this but, until recently, the Pill has been prescribed because HRT was not available in low enough doses to induce puberty (having been designed by drug companies for the older menopausal market).

There is an increasing debate about what type of medication to use as hormone replacement in girls with TS. Several British doctors argue that synthetic oestrogen (ethinyl oestradiol in tablets or combined with a progestogen in the contraceptive pill) is not the best choice because it can lead to inadvisable long-term use.[18] They point out that girls with TS often take the Pill for many years as adults simply because their prescriptions are not reviewed by specialists once they grow out of the UK adolescent health care system (and, in the UK National Health Service, the Pill is free of prescription charges, unlike HRT). They add that prolonged use of the Pill is associated with the risk of high blood pressure and blood clots; risks that are particularly unwelcome for women with TS as they are already prone to heart and blood pressure problems because of their condition. Long-term use of natural oestrogens found in some forms of HRT does not carry the same risks and is therefore seen as a better choice. The concern felt by these doctors is highlighted by recent data from 270 women aged 18–64 on the UK Turner Society register: 39 per cent were taking synthetic ethinyl oestradiol compared to 28 per cent using natural oestrogens.[19]

There is also an argument about when to begin hormone replacement and hence puberty in girls with TS. This is because a balance needs to be found between gaining height through growth hormone treatment and reaching puberty at a socially and psychologically acceptable age. Several researchers argue that oestrogen should be used so that girls with TS can go through puberty between 12 and 13 with their friends.[20] In contrast, one American doctor recommends that, after discussion with the patient and her family, oestrogen therapy and puberty should be delayed until age 14 onwards to allow growth hormone treatment to be completed beforehand and an improvement in final height.[21]

Several studies have highlighted the problems girls with TS can experience if they do not go through puberty with their friends. In particular, a recent Canadian study, based on in-depth interviews, found that women with TS often felt very isolated from their peers and family during adolescence, but that these feelings were far less intense or were absent in those who started on HRT aged 12–13.[22] As the researcher points out, the physical transformations that girls go through during puberty are given powerful social and psychological meanings. Against this backdrop, it isn't surprising that women in this study often described very painful feelings of being alone, different and 'less of a woman'.

The age at which girls with TS start hormone replacement has varied a lot, as data from 113 women in a current Australian study show: 3 per cent began before age 10; 30 per cent began between the ages of 11 and 15; 49 per cent began between 16 and 20 and 14 per cent began when they were over 21.[23] This can depend on when TS is diagnosed: nowadays girls are more likely to be diagnosed during childhood, rather than in their late teens because they lack their periods. Also, previous generations often received no or late HRT (see Bungy, Chapter 1), although this can still happen today.[24] For example, 4 per cent of the women in the Australian study had never received HRT and 17 per cent had stopped taking it, often below menopausal age and usually due to side-effects; 24 per cent of those on the UK Turner Society Register were not taking HRT.

Girls with androgen insensitivity syndrome can go through some of the outward signs of female puberty. This depends on whether their testes have been removed (gonadectomy or orchidectomy). AIS is often diagnosed because the testes cause inguinal hernias (bulging through the lower abdominal muscles) or because doctors find testes during an exploratory operation to investigate why a teenager hasn't started her periods. Doctors advise removing testes because they are associated with a 5–22 per cent risk of malignancy.[25] This estimate may be overstating the problem because AIS is rare and often undiagnosed due to secrecy. However, even an accurate estimate cannot predict *who* will develop malignancy, so while some women with AIS have kept their testes without difficulties, others developed malignancy and then had surgery. Where AIS can be diagnosed early because it runs in the family (22 per cent of cases), the testes may be removed while the child is very young (although this and any related genital plastic surgery can be controversial because the child cannot give consent.)[26]

Girls with AIS will develop breasts at puberty because some of their testosterone is converted by various tissues into oestrogen (see Figure 2.5, page 29). The reason that girls with AIS develop breasts and boys don't is probably because the oestrogen boys produce is balanced by their testosterone and related hormones (androgens).[27] Although girls with AIS produce these androgens, their cells can't receive the hormonal messages and so it is as if the hormones aren't present (just as during their development before birth). The result is that their oestrogen is never balanced as it is for boys and so girls with AIS develop breasts in much the same way as other women.

Lack of sensitivity to androgens also explains why girls with 'complete' AIS will not develop pubic or under-arm hair at puberty. Girls with 'partial' AIS can have pubic hair because they have some sensitivity to the androgens produced by their adrenal glands at this time. It is ironic that the existence of women without pubic hair has been ignored by Western society, while many a stone nymph displays her hairlessness in public parks and gardens, to say nothing of the nudes in old paintings who were brushed into decency. These bizarre contradictions would be laughable if teenagers and women with AIS had not dreaded discovery in school changing rooms or, later, by a potential partner.

Once girls and women with AIS have their testes removed, they need HRT like other young women without functioning ovaries. Since they do not have wombs, they are prescribed oestrogen-only HRT. That said, some doctors now advise starting oestrogen therapy in girls with AIS in late childhood (where diagnosed) because the body builds up the bones during puberty. For example, one research team suggests removing the testes at age 11 and slowly increasing the dose of oestrogen replacement while monitoring bone density.[28] They note that early treatment could be particularly important for girls with AIS because resistance to androgens in itself may affect bone building in early adolescence (although this requires further study).

However, puberty is not just about certain physical changes; it is also about developing sexuality. Women with TS, AIS and related conditions can have orgasms and positive sexual experiences (unless damaged by genital surgery), a view confirmed by some of the women who shared their experiences for this book. Nevertheless, these women can face very real practical problems. For example, vaginal dryness can be a worry for women with TS and others who have vaginas. This can be remedied in several ways (see Chapter 10) and often women feel more confident sexually as a result. If this isn't sufficient, women who are not androgen insensitive may find that testosterone replacement therapy helps their libido, although this is still experimental treatment and reports vary (see Jane, Chapter 1 and Juanita, below). Another problem may be lack of a full-length vagina. Vaginal dilation is described in Mary's story, below, and the use of oestrogen creams or pessaries can help this process in women with AIS. Further information on vaginal surgery (see Rosemary, Chapter 1 and Rosie, below) can be obtained through relevant support groups (see More Help).

Women with Turner syndrome, Swyer's syndrome or related conditions who have wombs can have children through egg donation and IVF. Although women with TS can need counselling about pregnancy, given the possible impact on any heart and kidney problems due to TS, research suggests that they are just as likely to get pregnant and carry the baby as other women undergoing egg donation. Egg-donation IVF is described in more detail in Chapter 7. There are other options such as adoption or surrogacy for all younger women with these conditions, whether they have a womb or not (see Mary, below).

Women's Stories

Joanne

I am 19 years old and have Turner's. I, like most other TS women, am on hormone replacement designed for post-menopausal women, Nuvelle to be exact. I am different from some women with TS in that I did have streak ovaries until I was about 14, when they disappeared, which the doctor who scanned me said would happen. This means I had the advantage of having some oestrogens for a little while.

I myself have had no medical problems relating to Turner's or HRT, apart from repetitive ear infections. I was on the Pill for a while, but then I was told that HRT would be better. There is a complete lack of information on this topic, which is relevant to women of my age. It is not helped by the fact that many of us, once we reach the age of about 16, are not seen by anyone other than our GPs to give us prescriptions.

Jennifer

I am 25 and studying for an MA in Librarianship. I am five foot tall. I was diagnosed as having Turner syndrome (TS) aged 11. I was told the full extent of TS six months later by my mother. I accepted the fact for better or worse, but realized that others would make it more of a problem than me and would never fully understand what it means to have this condition.

You are constantly told what is good for you and people talk down to or at you. Gaining control of your life and the condition is a struggle. Doctors' behaviour can be impersonal and overly clinical. This helps feed the idea, which you may already have, that you are somehow a second-class woman and deeply unfeminine. You have to develop independence and self-respect to survive and you definitely need a healthy scepticism towards the medical profession. I don't have a real problem with having TS, but doctors, the media and society want to push this unrealistic view of normality which excludes many people (not just women with TS).

I was put on a growth steroid for a year aged 12. When I was about 14, I was put on synthetic oestrogen. About a year later I was given progesterone. Both times I was very resentful. I thought I had escaped the horrors of puberty. To have things like periods, which would ultimately serve no purpose, as I then saw it, made me feel very uncomfortable. I have long since realized that to take oestrogen is the right thing as it is helpful psychologically to go through puberty (even if you do not realize it at the time).

At about 15 I was given the Pill by a specialist. I was deeply embarrassed about getting it from my local pharmacy. My 'well-informed' GP also asked why I was taking it and whether I was using it as a contraceptive! This is why I hated taking the Pill and why it is so inappropriate as a form of HRT. The Pill is used as HRT for young women in the UK, partly because it is free whereas HRT has to be paid for. I would rather pay than receive a free treatment that was inappropriate.

Aged 20, I participated in research on the effectiveness of HRT in building up bone in women with primary ovarian failure (especially TS). After discussing various forms of HRT, I went on Prempak-C. Although the doctor preferred implants, he let me choose and has always respected my decision. Thus I respect him! I discussed HRT with my aunt who is also taking it, as I had some reservations at first, but I feel I definitely made the right decision in swapping from the Pill. I find tablets are most convenient and give me most control (and that, for me, is most important). I can administer them myself and any problems are a lot easier to rectify than with, say, an implant.

But I still feel that once diagnosed as having TS you lose control over your body, no matter what way you choose to deal with it. You may have a say in your HRT, but you must take it in one form or another for a large part of your life or risk osteoporosis. I have seen the effects of osteoporosis and have no intention of getting it if I can help it.

I will have to take HRT for 30 years. I am not ecstatic about this. But I know the risks and I chose these over osteoporosis. One good thing about HRT is its beneficial effects on the heart and other areas.

I feel there are far worse medications to have to take for so long. It just requires education about the various forms of HRT, their benefits and drawbacks. However, you pretty much have to press doctors to get information and educate yourself to stay abreast of latest developments. I am also extremely concerned that we are the first group using HRT over such a long period. If there are drawbacks, they will show up in us and affect us the most.

Talking to others with TS, I have found HRT is very much 'horses for courses'. Some women like implants, some like patches or, like me, prefer tablets. I find talking with others very helpful; more helpful than talking to doctors, as women describe its effects (usually beneficial) a lot more clearly (or is it that I am far less sceptical about what they say?).

One thing really annoys me about the way doctors (often men) treat women with TS (and women generally!). We are expected to trust them, accept what they say and act on it. Where does this leave us when doctors say different things about HRT? Women with TS get caught in this cross-fire and can end up not knowing who to trust or what form of HRT to take. I know that most doctors do have the best interests of women with TS at heart and are trying to come to some sort of coherent policy.

Two things greatly anger me about the way HRT is talked about. Firstly, the media like to portray HRT as some luxury for post-menopausal women. They portray it in a flippant manner, downgrading it. They totally ignore its vital importance to women who, for whatever reason, have had an early menopause. They also jump on HRT scare stories for cheap sensationalism just as they jump on Pill scare stories. If HRT (or the Pill) was given to men, the products would be fully tested and there would be no such scare-mongering!

I also find the attitude of feminists who decry HRT deeply hypocritical. It is all very well for women who've benefited from two functioning ovaries for 30+ years to say eating fruit and drinking milk will get you over the menopause. What about those of us who have only had a few years – or even no years – of oestrogen to build up our bones! How is eating fruit going to help undo the damage an untreated premature menopause does to the body? I find that feminism has ignored women with TS or early menopause. It is a worthy movement, but it only really addresses itself to fertile women.

I would say (to paraphrase what the film-maker Derek Jarman said about having the HIV virus) that having TS and having to take HRT have been a gift that has enabled me to see things I would not have otherwise. I certainly find the friendship of other women with TS very rewarding.

Sherri Groveman (USA)

Several members of our support group have told me that they did not take HRT because it was a daily reminder of 'being different'. By not taking the pills, they could hide from having androgen insensitivity syndrome (AIS). I think the decision not to take HRT may be the only element of control they feel they have over a situation in which they largely feel a complete lack of control.

In my case, the ONLY thing my mother would ever mention about AIS – well, of course, she never actually told me I had AIS – so the only thing she would ever mention about my so-called 'twisted ovaries' was to ask if I was taking the pills. I was so angry at her for only being concerned about my physical welfare, and pretending there was no psychological trauma associated with all this, that I rebelled by not taking HRT. In an odd way, the pills became the embodiment of all my hurt, anger and frustration – as though the pills were the cause of my problem and without the pills the problem would just go away.

Moreover, my mother made me go to the pharmacy to have the HRT prescription filled. I was consumed with fear that the pharmacist knew something was terribly wrong with me, and that by just presenting the prescription he would know exactly what that something was (I didn't understand at the time – about age 11 – that there were many reasons why someone took Premarin – I thought it was a specific drug for my own condition, so that by looking at the prescription, the pharmacist would know I had 'twisted ovaries', couldn't have children, didn't have pubic hair, etc.).

As I got a bit older and understood that 'old' ladies took Premarin as hormone replacement, I felt equally embarrassed that I, as a teenager, had a prescription for the same drug. I knew that even if women in their thirties had hysterectomies and needed HRT, it was still grotesquely abnormal for a 12–13-year-old to be turning up with a prescription for it.

I was also terrified to carry the pills in my purse for fear of discovery. When I was in college, I was afraid to even have them in my dorm room for fear one of my friends would stumble across them while looking for something else. It was about this time that I stopped taking HRT altogether. Whereas my mother dragged me to the reproductive endocrinologist as a teenager, once I was on my own, I just couldn't summon up the strength and courage to locate and be examined by another doctor, which was a requirement if I was going to get replacement prescriptions for HRT.

I have spent a great deal of time in therapy discussing and crying over the trauma of being on HRT at an early age. I cry over the fact that at a time of life when all my friends got their periods, I instead got a pill. I didn't want 'womanhood from a bottle'. I desperately wanted to cross the threshold into womanhood in the same way as my friends did – by having a menstrual cycle. When I resumed HRT in my thirties (I stopped taking it from 17 until 35), it was a cathartic moment to walk into a pharmacy and hand the prescription to the person behind the counter. It brought back a flood of memories.

Rosie

I am in my forties and have androgen insensitivity syndrome (AIS). At birth I appeared to be a normal baby girl, but I have always suspected my biological mix-up. About aged 10, my parents told me that the scars in my groin were from a hernia operation when I was a toddler and that the surgeon had said that I would probably not menstruate or be able to have children. After secretly looking in a medical dictionary, I realized that hernias were something odd which girls didn't have. Soon after this, I checked and discovered my absent vagina but was too frightened to mention this to anyone. I decided that I had no chance of having relationships or ever getting married.

I remember my best friend having her period while staying at my house and feeling very excluded. Not having the bother or cramps is no comfort whatsoever compared to the immense reassurance I would have had of an essential femaleness. The other sign of femininity, breast development, didn't happen until very late and I was petrified in the changing rooms of being seen to have no pubic hair (a feature of my condition). I felt that I must be fundamentally male and this worried me intensely, but I kept this to myself, having absorbed the atmosphere of secrecy during visits to the family GP, who would always say, 'Let's leave it until she's a bit older and see what happens.' I was 18 before the medical profession caught up with things.

A local gynaecologist confirmed my worst fears and told me to come back for plastic surgery *if I wanted to get married*. He 'explained' that a surgically created vagina would probably close up if I wasn't having regular sex – and I got the strong message that I was not entitled to treatment unless I was. The non-surgical 'do-it-yourself' method of vaginal pressure dilation (which has been around since 1938) was not – and never has been – mentioned. But he added optimistically that there was no reason not to regard myself as 'a perfectly normal female'. This seemed like telling someone with no legs to come back when they could walk to see if artificial limbs could be fitted to enable them to run, but that in the meantime there was no reason not to consider herself to be an athlete. And how was I going to meet a partner when I dreaded anyone knowing of my situation?

It felt hopeless. I couldn't press for surgery without the established boyfriend because they would think I wanted to be promiscuous. Couldn't they see that this was all too much for me to bring up on my own – and that I was far too traumatized and intimidated to say anything to this middle-aged man in a shiny brown suit behind a mahogany desk who had just confirmed that I had XY chromosomes, abdominal testes and no vagina? Why was no one volunteering to help me? I wanted some kindly 'auntie' to sweep in and say, 'Yes, you're entitled to share your life with someone, let's see what we can do to make that possible.' Instead I felt everyone had given up on me because I was such a freak and not entitled to any sort of sexuality. I was too embarrassed to ask for counselling and the situation has never been discussed in my family.

The truth hurts, no matter how one finds it out, but the pain is not in the shock of hearing about a small piece of DNA or the nature of a bundle of cells in one's abdomen. It is in the prospect of living your entire life with so many questions and anxieties about who you are and your hopes of getting close to other people, while feeling too afraid to ever *imagine* saying this to anyone and thus getting help.

After my testes were removed when I was 24, I had an oestrogen implant, then later I was prescribed ethinyl oestradiol tablets. However, they caused side-effects and enlarged my breasts, so I felt better when I stopped taking them and never had hot flushes (unlike some women with AIS). I was delighted when I was prescribed the Pill as HRT instead and had those dinky packets with days of the month on them. I could kind of pretend I was normal and had a sex life, etc.

However, by 28, my self-confidence was at rock bottom. I hadn't even been able to tell a female friend that I couldn't have children, never mind anything else, and I feared being drawn into discussing periods, babies, sex and relationships. And because my worst nightmare was a partner finding out that I couldn't have sex, I shrank from even superficial social encounters for fear of where they might lead.

Eventually I decided to ask the local gynaecologist to operate. This didn't have a great deal to do with sex; I just wanted to feel that I had the same basic equipment as other women for my own peace of mind, even if I never found a boyfriend. I was too frightened to seek out, say, a London specialist with perhaps more expertise because I had never voluntarily brought up my condition in front of another human being. The surgery was a complete waste of time. The vagina shrank almost to its pre-op length, so I was still no nearer being a 'normal woman'. I suffered a lot and was left with a 5" × 7" scar at the site of the donor skin graft – yet another thing to explain.

Over the next 10 years I had a few approaches, but I rejected them at the outset, knowing that we couldn't go anywhere and dreading having to reveal things. A female doctor then became the first person to encourage me to seek treatment even though I didn't have a boyfriend, referring me to a gynaecologist who suggested a different surgical procedure. It sounded highly complex and not quite like a proper vagina. Was it worth the physical and emotional pain, and would more surgery fix the way I felt about myself? All I wanted was what other women take for granted. It didn't seem like a lot to ask. Yet medical science was too busy advancing fertility treatment for women already a million miles ahead of me in their expression of femaleness. I let the offer slip.

Then I met someone special. We were so well matched and both wanted a physical relationship. I panicked and asked for surgery, but there was a 10-month waiting list. By the time I had the op, he had cooled off. We only had sex once or twice – essentially the relationship was over before it had started. I blurted out the whole story; he admitted that the new vagina was too short (he was actually quite large) and then freaked out at my revelation and disappeared into the sunset. This was probably largely due to the terrible state I was in whilst telling him – having never practised the words with someone 'safe'. I was totally devastated. It could have been my only chance of a partnership and I hadn't been able to prepare myself.

Since then I have had another relationship, but the physical side hasn't worked out and I have not been able to bring myself to tell him anything about my situation. I feel a conflict between the desire to pass as a normal woman with a man (with a reluctance to risk destroying the 'illusion') and the wish to experience his reaction to the truth (in the desperate hope that it will not make any difference).

Looking back, I feel that most of the damage was done during my teens when I waited, knowing I had a problem, until doctors clarified it but then offered no resolution. Although I never wanted to be other than a woman, I wasn't sure whether others saw me as truly female and so did not have a clear sense of what and who I was. Counselling and being put in touch with others with AIS when I was younger might have prevented this. The problems of developing any sort of sexuality and partnership have meant that infertility has been a distant issue for me. Knowing that I would never form part of the obligatory couple meant I never allowed myself the luxury of imagining I might care for adopted or surrogate children. HRT has been even more distant. I have tried various types of Pill, Premarin, Livial (tibolone), natural progesterone, Progynova TS (patch) and even testosterone. However, for many years I only took HRT intermittently and I now have significant osteoporosis. Oestrogen cannot give me female internal organs or pubic hair or a proper vagina and its supposed health benefits (heart, bones) seem remote compared to what I've lived with since childhood.

Juanita (USA)

I was diagnosed with Swyer's syndrome at 17 when I failed to menstruate. My doctor said the procedure for my condition was to remove the streak gonads and part of the Fallopian tubes. During surgery he found a tumour on the gonadal tissue and chose to perform a complete hysterectomy. Apparently my uterus was very underformed and he felt the tumour could have been malignant. It ended up being benign. A percentage of Swyer's women are prone to developing this type of dysgerminoma [early tumour]. If they don't, only the gonadal tissue is removed and the uterus remains. In my case, the results of Swyer's have been no menstruation and infertility.

I began taking oestrogen (Premarin 1.25 mg) and progesterone (Provera 2.5 mg). At first I took it on a cycle: Premarin and Provera on days 1–25 and then five days off. I was told Provera was primarily for breast development. In the first year my breasts developed somewhat. They are small, but before surgery they had been non-existent as I was pre-pubescent until I began HRT.

I continued on this hormone regime for six years when I felt the cyclical nature of the routine wasn't working for me. I felt the five days off were making me physically depressed. So my doctor recommended both hormones continuously. This seemed to help.

At 27, I began graduate studies at a large university with an excellent health clinic linked to a research hospital. My new doctor recommended I stop the progesterone as my breasts would not develop any further. So I continued with oestrogen only.

By then, I had dated occasionally but not had intercourse. During graduate school I entered into my first committed relationship. My boyfriend was very understanding about my lack of sexual experience and so I felt I could 'learn' with him. We chose not to have intercourse for a variety of reasons. However, our petting, and at times heavy petting, brought up psychological issues surrounding my sexuality.

I began to see a psychiatrist at the health clinic. As we talked about my relationship, my sexual history, my virginity, he asked if I had ever had my androgen levels checked. I said I had no idea what he was talking about. So he conferred with my gynaecologist and she also recommended my levels being checked.

The results of this blood test showed I had no free androgens in my system. My psychiatrist explained that androgens, mainly testosterone, can correlate with libido and that women as well as men produce them. He recommended that I consider supplementing my HRT with testosterone.

I was shocked yet intrigued by the possibility of testosterone HRT. Would this sexual drive I never had now be available to me? I waited a few months to try testosterone for fear my newly found libido might rage during my intense school schedule, leaving me running through the streets after any available man. However, as I began to take the new hormone, I found the process to be one of gradual awareness. The best way I can describe it is as a sort of awakening. I began to have sexual dreams about men, which I had had only intermittently before. The old dreams were more about an emotional connection than a sexual one. For example, I would see a man, be attracted to him and he would put his arm around me and I would feel connected to him. However, my new dreams contained kissing and fondling and I could now see naked bodies and penises, even erect ones. In my waking life, I began to feel a new awareness of sexual attraction, noticing men in a more sexual way than I had before. Interestingly my relationship with my boyfriend began to taper off. I didn't tell him I was now taking testosterone. I was scared to. We broke up a few months later when I moved to a new city.

I was told testosterone can also be correlated with attention span and mental sharpness. As I began my new HRT, I felt I had a greater ability to connect ideas and follow a more complex train of thought. I also felt able to entertain a more mature thought process. In short, I felt as if I was going through puberty at 29. It took about two and a half years to get the dosage level correct on my testosterone (see page 225). Now, with my doctor's support, I use a pill-splitting device to take *half* the Estratest HS dose (i.e. 0.625 mg testosterone/0.31 mg oestrogen) and 0.9 mg Premarin to make up my oestrogen to 1.21 mg.* This seems right for me.

I'd like to say that I'm now sexually active but I'm not. Sometimes, most times, this embarrasses me and I rarely discuss it outside of close family and friends. When women start swapping stories about their sexual escapades, I sit quietly and listen and try to laugh and nod at the appropriate times, pretending that I know exactly what they're talking about when I don't. I feel now that I'm much closer to trusting a man with my body, but it's taken me quite some time to adjust to this new hormone inside of me as well as deal with the shame I've felt about my condition; no menstruation, infertility and, well, puberty quite delayed.

I do masturbate occasionally. At first this was an important way for me to connect to my body and my sexuality, to know that my body does respond to sexual stimulation, to be able to experience that sensation, to know my body can have pleasure. However, now masturbating often leaves me feeling depressed for I do long for a partner and stimulating myself isn't enough after all.

In general, my body awareness is improving, though. While I have a fairly trim body, I often hide it under formless clothing. Most recently a friend advised getting in touch with my hips by taking a dance class. I have realized that because my lower regions are infertile and lack menstruation, I have wanted to ignore them. There is no

* Estratest is not available in the UK at the time of writing.

biological clock ticking, as it were, no pendulum swaying, moving hips to and fro in a hypnotic motion to capture the heart of some forthright young man. But I am realizing that I can move them myself and connect to them on my own.

So testosterone has given me this new awakening, this new chapter in my physical recovery. The potential negative side-effects are hirsutism and liver-function damage. The level I take is said to be safe for the liver, although my doctor has me take a liver-function test every six months.* I do have more hair than before and I'm not sure if it is due to the sole influence of the hormone or if I've simply come from a genetically hairy family. It's nothing dramatic and ape-like (which was my fear), just more than I had before.

Taking testosterone also coincided with a new level of awareness about my condition. I asked to go over my initial medical records with my doctor. I had known the basic details of my condition, but I had no comprehension of the genetics issue. When my psychiatrist finally explained it to me, my first reaction was fear. I tried to talk to some close friends about it and got a mixed response. It wasn't until I joined the AIS Support Group that I was able to gain greater self-acceptance. I came to understand that the genetic component was really inconsequential for me. It was a genetic event that had occurred during pregnancy and once the foetus had formed as female, the XY issue was over. I am fully female.

I think the hardest side of all this has been slowly crawling out of puberty and realizing how much of a girl/woman I have been for so long. Sexuality has been scary for me. While people tell me I'm attractive, I have felt very vulnerable about attracting men and being sexual. I originally feared a man would reject me because I couldn't conceive or because I was a virgin or simply because I was 'different'. I no longer have these fears as much. I guess I have the knowledge now that none of that really matters when it comes to a relationship for me. I need to be with a man who will accept me as I am.

As for infertility, I share this experience with many women and so

---

* This is unlikely to be available routinely in the UK.

I don't feel so alone in that. The lack of menstruation, never having had that rite of passage, is hard at times. I often feel like I'm on a different wavelength from other women – and in some ways I am. I just don't have the hormonal swings and that drive-for-sex-so-I-can-reproduce element.

So at 32 I'm on a different path than most women I meet. It comforts me to know there are other women on a similar path for other reasons, that I am not alone in being infertile, lacking menstruation and sexual experience at my age. However, I will always be 'out of sync' with many women. Through the effects of my HRT, talking to others with similar conditions, talking to family and close friends about my truth and through my own writing about all of this, I am learning to accept myself more and more. I find one positive result of my condition is that I have a greater focus and portion of energy to devote to my work as a writer – that my female creativity has an outlet here and that my female identity is so much more than my lack of reproductive organs.

Mary

When young deaf children draw self-portraits they often draw a face framed by exceedingly large ears. My picture would show a round tummy with a big hole in it.

My story begins when I was about 13 and, like most teenagers, wanted an excuse not to have a communal shower after sport at school. But there were no excuses, *everyone had* to have a shower . . . unless you looked earnest and whispered it was 'that time of the month'. Then you'd get a sympathetic nod and remain nice and sweaty for the rest of the day. So that's what I did, every few weeks, and carried it off well. I also managed to sit through embarrassingly long conversations about periods, sanitary towels, tampons, sex and more, and none of my friends ever suspected a thing. But the truth was I hadn't started my periods – and never have since. The only difference now is that I don't pretend any more. Since my twenties, if the subject comes up with new friends, my lack of periods is envied rather than pitied. I know other young women without periods like me feel regret, but I've never missed or ever really wanted periods, not even during the heady days of school.

My story, however, is not simply about a lack of menstrual blood every month. By 16 I was physically developed in all other ways, a successful student and athlete, not unattractive and content in close friendships, but I began to realize that something was wrong. All girls investigate themselves and I was tame about it, but when I did I became very confused. My earliest recollections are of fear of intercourse because I just couldn't comprehend how one did it. I also worried about what I'd do with tampons if I ever needed one. Because there is so much secrecy about what I have now learnt is my condition, I was very alone with my fears at this time. After all, sex education never taught you there could possibly be a situation like mine. So I comforted myself by thinking all girls were like me, and that's why your 'first time' hurt. I steered well clear of over-keen boyfriends. As far as I could work out, it could only be absolute agony.

My Mum and I went to the doctor about my periods, but were always sent off with a 'not to worry' diagnosis. At 16 this changed. I was sent to a gynaecologist who said I needed an exploratory operation (laparoscopy). As we were leaving, he whispered to my Mum not to feel 'too hopeful'. I assumed I wasn't ever going to start my periods; anything else was outside my conscious thoughts. I think it must have been outside my parents' too. I have a very close relationship with my Mum and I'm sure I *would* have asked her, but if you don't know a condition exists, then, I guess, there's nothing to ask.

I went into hospital for my laparoscopy. The next day, the consultant decided to treat me like an adult and give me the results without informing my parents. That is what he told me, anyway. Probably he was in a hurry. But the enormity of his news was too much for a 16-year-old to hear alone. He drew some diagrams, gave me the facts and was gone, leaving me to phone my parents, begging them to come quick.

To be fair, this consultant gave me the fullest explanation I've ever received and the only knowledge I had for the next 15 years. He said

I had two working ovaries but no womb and because my womb hadn't developed I had no vagina, as this normally drops down from the womb. I couldn't have children and, unless I had an operation (which wasn't always successful), I wouldn't have sexual intercourse either. And finally I probably only had one kidney (later tests confirmed this), which is OK as we only need one anyway. I can so clearly remember his drawing with two egg sacks dropping eggs into empty space. Even now I have visions of lost eggs wandering around inside me with nowhere to go. I can see the one lonely kidney he drew and that was it. There was nothing else on the paper. That was the hole in my tummy I've been carrying around ever since.

I don't know how I coped emotionally during the following weeks. I think the double blow of not being able to have intercourse *or* children was too much and I suppressed thoughts about children until later years. At this stage, I was more concerned about my vagina (or lack of it). We decided to see a specialist about the operation after my exams. I remember talking to some close friends, who were very sympathetic and understanding, but also rather horrified and determined that I should get something done quickly. My parents told me we would do all we could to sort this out, even if that meant sending me to America. An old boyfriend who'd become a medical student said he'd research what could be done. So from the beginning it was fully assumed I had a big 'problem' which should be put right.

Against this background, I went to see a top gynaecologist. I was quite excited. After all, this was a special appointment at a hospital far from home, which offered the prospect of making me more 'normal', and this could only be good. All I can say is that this visit left me in such shock that even thinking about it now, 15 years later, is difficult. I consider myself strong emotionally, but I still cannot go near that hospital.

It's hard to explain why it was so horrendous. Basically there I was, a 17-year-old girl who was weighed, measured, told to get undressed and left to wait alone in a Spartan cubicle. My mother was somehow sidelined to wait elsewhere. I had no idea what would happen. Suddenly the curtain was pulled back and there seemed to be about 10 people in white coats standing around the bed. What appeared to me to be a very old man barked at me to lie in a foetal position and when I did so, he lifted my gown and began to explain to his entourage exactly what was wrong with me. I felt completely humiliated as he poked about with all these eyes glaring down upon this 'rarity'. He then announced he would perform the operation by taking a skin graft from my leg to create a false vagina and were there any questions? I think I asked if it would leave a scar on my leg, was told probably a little one, and then he and his followers were gone. He didn't even ask if a parent was present, which made my mother furious.

I remember crying with my Mum outside the hospital and vowing I would never let that man near my body again and to hell with this operation for the time being. This decision, taken in shock, turned out to be one of the best of my life. I was lucky. My parents supported whatever decision I made. I reacted adversely to being treated like a scientific lump of meat on a table. I was exposed as a freak who had to be put right: given a vagina. There was no other way of being normal. I hope that nowadays girls in this vulnerable position are approached with incredible sensitivity and given more options.

I want to mention one disturbing repercussion caused by my absent vagina that, in retrospect, was compounded by being treated like a 'freak'. Soon after diagnosis I had recurrent nightmares about rape. I had visions of a rapist attacking me and discovering my 'abnormality'; his manhood being violated and the attack then becoming even more violent and grotesque. Other women like me have similar nightmares; it appears to be a common psychological effect of our condition.

Soon after my awful consultation I passed my exams and had a year out before university. During that time I met my first real boyfriend and he was absolutely wonderful about everything. I decided to approach men with the attitude that it was their problem if they couldn't handle the situation. My mother says she hasn't forgotten the day I said, soon after my diagnosis, that at least I would know that if a man was to love me, then it really would be *me* he loved. I can honestly say that the men I have told have always been amazingly understanding. Because I have a clitoris and can have an orgasm, I can also have good sexual relationships without intercourse (although doctors never gave me such information or reassurance). I am indebted to this first lover for teaching me that and giving me so much confidence.

None the less, after my degree, I did feel ready to re-investigate what could be done about my vagina. I went to a women's hospital, assuming the consultant would talk about surgery. I still felt incredibly anxious about an operation. Somehow it felt like a violation of my body. I hated the idea of a skin graft and couldn't envisage how a vagina could be created without it being incredibly painful, inefficient and solely there to satisfy a man sexually. I was overjoyed when the consultant recommended vaginal dilators.

With the dilation method you create a vagina by exerting pressure on the skin covering where the vagina should be. If this is successful, the skin slowly stretches upwards. As the space gets bigger, the doctor issues a larger dilator and so on. In very successful cases you eventually build an almost normal-sized opening. As I walked out of the hospital, I remember feeling incredibly excited and eager to start immediately. Armed with my tiny dilator, I shut myself in my bedroom and set to work. It wasn't particularly painful, but it wasn't easy at first. However, I was amazed at how quickly the hole increased. I think the consultant was too.

I turned out to be a real success story! Several months later I moved south, began my first job and met my future husband. The timing could not have been better. The consultant had said a sexual partner would really help and she was correct. Soon I was able to have intercourse for the first time. And to my pleasant surprise the whole process had been well worth it and love-making was extremely satisfying for us both. My partner says my vagina feels very normal and because I created it in what I see as a 'natural' way, it also feels very much part of me. I quite like the way its size changes depending on how sexually active I am. That's me now.

I still feel an operation would have left me feeling intruded upon, as if something had been stitched to my body that wasn't really supposed to be there and that, if I didn't like it, could never be taken away. People's immediate reflex that a false vagina must be created surgically is, I feel, an attitude left over from the past, when sex was seen as something to satisfy men, intercourse was the only meaningful sexual activity and reproduction was the main aim. I know that for a lot of women without a vagina, surgery is sometimes the only option and I often wonder what I would have done had this been the case for me. However, I also know that now it is more common to try dilators first. It makes me smile even as I write this when I think how fortunate I was to walk away from that horrendous consultant at 17.

The other problems that emerged during these years were hormonal. My doctor assumed I had hormonal cycles, but had no real proof of this. Until about 21 I didn't have symptoms that suggested a cycle, but then I began to get water retention, which lasted for weeks, months, getting worse until I felt I was going to explode. My breasts were exceedingly tender. I tried various remedies, but nothing helped until my body adjusted itself. My doctors agreed I might be experiencing a massive build-up of oestrogen and gave me danazol, a drug which reduces female hormones. I was so ecstatic about solving my problem that I didn't question how strong this drug might be or its long list of side-effects. Only in recent years have I found out how important adequate oestrogen is in terms of osteoporosis.

As years have gone by and I have less water retention, and hence less indication of my fluctuating oestrogen, I have become concerned about premature menopause and osteoporosis. I put all this to my doctor and she agreed it was certainly an area for concern; she arranged a hormone blood test and agreed it would be sensible to carry out this test annually. My results were normal and it is comforting to know that, at 32, I don't have to worry about HRT just yet!

About five years ago, I tried to find out if I was fertile as my partner and I were investigating ways of starting a family and dabbled with the idea of surrogacy. My doctor suggested using a temperature fertility chart to see if I had a monthly peak. I persevered, but I had absolutely no pattern at all. Although this wasn't conclusive, we decided against further tests to check my fertility and began an assessment for adoption. This was very challenging emotionally and my grief about my inability to have children by birth bubbled to the surface and has stayed for the time being. This is ironic as we have now adopted the most wonderful boy, who we couldn't possibly love any more if he'd been born from my body 10 times over. We are also about to embark on a second adoption.

I think what keeps my grief lingering is the fact that adoption is clearly a very different process from childbirth and it throws up problems that never go away, like the fact that our son will always have his 'birth family' and his 'real' mum (as everyone always refers to the birth mother). He'll have many emotional bridges to cross in his life regarding his roots and his adoptive family. I worry about these and how he'll cope and, yes, how I'll cope. I guess what I really really want is for our son to be exactly the way he is – for I wouldn't want him any other way – but to have come out of my body, so that we could erase any emotional confusion in years to come. In a way these are selfish thoughts and I don't have them often, but I don't deny they exist and that they will always be part of a grieving process for different elements of my lost 'womanhood'.

If there was ever to be an end to this story, it would probably come now. I am happily married with a gorgeous son and we may be able to complete our family with a second adoption. However, since discovering the AIS Support Group and meeting women in similar situations, I realize my search to understand everything that has happened and is happening is only really beginning. What I've done for 15 years is live with and cope with my condition. Until four months ago, I didn't even have a name for it. Now I know it is called Mayer-Rokitansky-Kuster-Hauser (MRKH) syndrome; however ridiculous a title, it would have been good to know the name from Day 1. It gives an identity that is important to me. For a very long time, I've been told that I was just 'born that way' as others are born without arms or legs. This limited sort of explanation seems to be a way of maintaining the veil of secrecy which surrounds these sexual conditions. At no point has any doctor suggested putting me in touch with other women; at no point did anyone suggest that I might benefit from some counselling. I have only ever been sent away with the feeling that it's best to keep quiet and get on with life.

I have been exceedingly lucky: I am emotionally strong, I've had a very supportive family and I've been attracted to men who, even if they couldn't handle the situation, were none the less very polite and let me walk away feeling this was their inadequacy rather than mine. I grew up with what I see as progressive ideas on sexuality and sexual relationships. I met a man who, as I predicted all those years ago, really loves me for who I am and we are managing to bring children into our lives and gain incredible pleasure as a family. I often wonder with horror what would have happened to women with MRKH syndrome during the last century and before. I wonder about women in other cultures where sexual issues are even more taboo. But, perhaps because it is closest to home, I think most about teenage girls being diagnosed now. I want to help ensure that they do not have to wait for support. No one should be alone with these conditions.

7

PREMATURE MENOPAUSE

'It was the very invisibility of premature menopause that caused the problems. Those close to me took the doctor's view that, apart from infertility, I was a "perfectly normal young woman". There was no breakdown, no real illness in evidence Just the slow chipping away at my self-image.'

SUSAN

The menopause occurs when the ovaries run out of follicles. Usually this takes place mid-life, but it can happen almost any time earlier. In fact, premature menopause is surprisingly common. According to an American study, 1 in every 1000 women will have spontaneous ovarian failure before the age of 30.[1] This statistic rises to 1 in every 100 women by the time they reach 40. These estimates do not include younger women who have a surgical or medical menopause.

When their ovaries fail unexpectedly, women want to know why. In most cases doctors won't know the answer; medical understanding of this condition is itself rather young. For example, premature ovarian failure (POF) was only formally defined in 1967 and research has intensified rather more recently. This is partly because it has taken time for researchers to develop ways of measuring relevant hormones and arrive at a more detailed understanding of the menstrual cycle and ovarian follicles (see Chapter 2).

This chapter looks at what happens when women have a spontaneous premature menopause, whether in their teens, twenties or thirties. It describes how ovarian failure is diagnosed, why a younger woman may lack follicles and the options for fertility treatment. Women who have had the shock of a premature menopause tell their stories. Some also speak about their experiences of egg-donation IVF (in-vitro fertilization).

Getting a Diagnosis

Like the natural menopause, a premature menopause may not lead to hot flushes and night sweats. According to one study, only 50 per cent of women with premature ovarian failure have these signs.[2] Even if younger women have menopausal symptoms they tend to explain them away, only later realizing their significance. Many women delay visiting their doctors until their periods go awry and there is no obvious explanation, such as pregnancy.

Research to date suggests that, on average, women with premature ovarian failure start their periods in the same way and at about the same time as other women.[3] In general, they have a normal menstrual cycle until their problems arise. Then their periods may become few and far between or stop suddenly. Some women find their natural periods never return when they come off the Pill, an experience which can lead to understandably shocked regret (see Pippa, below). In some cases this may be due to an upset in the hypothalamus rather than the ovaries.

Women can miss their periods for all sorts of 'everyday' reasons (see Figure 7.1) and so GPs are often slow to take the possibility of premature menopause seriously. For example, one study found that 9 out of 10 young women with missing periods lack them for other reasons, a finding that fits most GPs' experience.[4] This means that GPs may suggest waiting for several months to see if periods return before conducting hormone tests.

Doctors often start by measuring blood levels of FSH. The reason for this may not be obvious. After all, why not measure oestrogen, the hormone that women are said to lack after the menopause? The answer is that blood oestradiol levels do not necessarily *warn* of ovarian failure. As described in Chapter 3, FSH tends to rise in the run-up to a woman's final period, whereas oestradiol falls to a

Figure 7.1 *Some* reasons why younger women can lack periods

1 'Obvious' reasons, e.g. pregnancy, lack of ovaries or lack of womb or vagina (see Chapter 6).

2 Disruption of the hormonal messages that control the menstrual cycle caused by problems in the hypothalamus or pituitary gland. This may be due to 'everyday' reasons (e.g. being very under- or overweight) or, less commonly, to intensive sports training, previous use of the contraceptive pill, a benign pituitary tumour, etc.

3 Disruption caused by ovarian failure due to:
   • Lack of egg-containing follicles and their ability to produce hormones, often for unknown reasons or perhaps due to genetic problems that interrupted ovarian development before birth (see also Chapter 6).*
   • Damage to the supply of follicles; may be obvious damage caused by surgery (surgical menopause) or radio/chemotherapy (medical menopause) or supposed damage, perhaps due to auto-immune problems, etc.

4 Present but unresponsive ovarian follicles (resistant ovary syndrome).

* This can lead to early loss of periods, but if the lack of follicles is acute, then girls cannot produce all the hormones needed for puberty and to begin menstruation. Women who never have periods may be told they have primary amenorrhoea (whereas women whose periods begin but later stop unexpectedly have secondary amenorrhoea). Amenorrhoea simply means absence of monthly flow.

suspiciously low level at a later stage. Therefore high FSH levels can be a sign that the pituitary is trying to kick-start failing ovaries.

However, in the absence of symptoms, a 'high FSH' result can be deceiving for several reasons. Firstly, women vary. Secondly, FSH also rises before ovulation, although to a lesser extent. This means that doctors may have to check whether they are looking at a FSH rise due to ovulation *or* ovarian failure. They can do this by repeating the blood test to see whether the FSH level has dropped or not. Premature ovarian failure is suspected if FSH remains unexpectedly high in a woman under the age of 40 without periods. What counts as 'unexpectedly high' depends on the laboratory doing the test and the doctor interpreting the result. Most doctors become suspicious if the level remains in double figures. Researchers' definitions vary from above 20 iu/l[5] to above 30 iu/l[6] or above 40 iu/l.[7]

This lack of a clear 'yes' result can seem odd when compared to tests such as the pregnancy test. However, the pregnancy test measures a hormone that only appears during pregnancy and is detectable within weeks of conceiving, i.e. either one is pregnant or not. In contrast, ovarian failure is a slow process of hormonal change from normal to menopausal, which may not be easy to identify or measure until later. This means doctors often have to judge FSH levels against other signs and symptoms to arrive at a diagnosis. Usually they are looking for an overall *trend* rather than a single test result. In other words, FSH numbers aren't everything!

Even when the diagnosis seems clear, doctors can be proved wrong because the pituitary manages to get the ovary going again. Women have been known to ovulate later in spite of an apparent menopause and, very occasionally, such women have become pregnant without fertility treatment (see Pip, Chapter 1). FSH levels cannot predict who might be surprised by a recovery,[8] although this is thought to be very unlikely in women with repeated FSH measurements above 100 iu/l.[9]

When trying to reach a diagnosis, doctors may check several other hormones, including thyroid hormones and the pituitary hormones LH and prolactin. The thyroid controls the body's metabolism and sometimes correcting this can restore menstruation, although thyroid problems are also associated with ovarian failure (see Monique, below). LH levels rise after the menopause, so levels that remain unexpectedly high can provide another reason to suspect ovarian failure. This seems straightforward, but why check prolactin, the hormone for breast milk?

The answer is clearer when one remembers that regular breastfeeding can delay the return of women's periods. High prolactin levels switch off the menstrual cycle, and with good reason, after pregnancy, as they can help women avoid renewed fertility at a demanding time for their bodies. However, prolactin levels can rise at other times, perhaps because of stress or as a side-effect of certain drugs. Occasionally the reason is a benign pituitary tumour (adenoma).

Small benign pituitary tumours are quite common and may never cause any trouble, but they can lead to lack of periods. Doctors can be confused by this because the FSH test gives a normal or low result in this case.[10] Yet repeated prolactin tests will show high levels and provide the clue that further investigations are needed, such as an MRI scan. If the problem lies simply in the pituitary, then treatment will help the patient ovulate and restore her hormone levels (or she can be given HRT).

Looking for Follicles

High FSH levels suggest that the pituitary is trying to stimulate the ovaries, but this finding does not tell doctors whether this is because of a lack of follicles (a true menopause) or unresponsive follicles (resistant ovary syndrome). Nothing can be done about absent follicles, but 'resistant' follicles may be persuaded to release their eggs – at least, in theory.

In the past, doctors looked for signs of follicles by doing an ovarian biopsy, which involves removing a piece of tissue for examination. However, such surgery did not necessarily increase doctors' ability to predict a woman's chances of pregnancy or alter the recommended treatment. In short, it wasn't clear whether the supposed difference between premature menopause and resistant ovary syndrome was meaningful.

Today doctors check women's ovaries using an ultrasound scan. This type of scan builds up a picture using the echoes of sound waves, rather like a sonar. If this makes one think of water, then it won't be too surprising to hear that this is one of the reasons why women are asked to fill their bladders before a conventional abdominal scan. Not only does a full bladder push the bowel out of the way, but 'water' improves the clarity of the picture. The image is obtained by passing a probe across the abdomen or, more occasionally, placing it within the vagina (on an empty bladder). A vaginal probe gets closer to the ovaries, which may be an advantage in this case as women with ovarian failure can have small ovaries. However, some researchers think that smaller ovaries are easier to detect with an abdominal scan.[11] Either way, ovaries can prove hard to find among the pelvic organs.

Ovarian follicles may show up on an ultrasound scan as dark areas against the ovarian tissue. Different studies have reported follicles in 16, 20 and 50 per cent of women with premature ovarian failure using ultrasound.[12] Yet another study found follicles in 60 per cent of those investigated.[13] This range of findings suggests either that the presence of follicles varies a lot or that some researchers have better detection rates, or both. A scan is only a 'snapshot' of what may be happening on the ovaries at a given moment, and not a very clear one at that. Still, techniques are improving all the time, so perhaps follicles are present far more often than previously thought? This returns us to the question of whether there is a true difference between premature menopause (apparent lack of follicles) and resistant ovary syndrome (unresponsive follicles). So far no one really knows. The answer matters because if doctors get better at finding supposedly absent follicles, then this raises the possibility that patients may conceive – or be helped to conceive – with their own eggs in future.

Some researchers think that resistant ovary syndrome is due to a lack of FSH receptors on the follicle, although others believe that it has more to do with oestrogen receptors because a few patients receiving HRT have recovered their ability to ovulate and even become pregnant.[14] This is a hopeful sign that the problem may be reversible in future, although so far doctors have been frustrated in most of their attempts to perform such miracles to order.

Why Younger Women Can Lack Follicles

A baby's ovaries store eggs in follicles before birth. This supply cannot be renewed, so, if development is interrupted, the baby will be born with ovaries that contain fewer follicles. A small reserve may lead to a lack of puberty or periods followed by an unwelcome premature menopause, depending on how long her supply lasts. Alternatively a girl can be born with plenty of follicles, but there may be a problem with her menopausal 'body-clock'. This clock times the follicle 'clearout' that takes place before the natural menopause. In some cases, this may be triggered earlier than usual. Lastly, she may have a plentiful supply of follicles that is damaged for some reason, causing premature ovarian failure.

Sometimes women's lack of follicles can be explained by a genetic problem such as a missing, damaged or extra X chromosome that interrupts ovarian development (see also Chapter 6). However, relatively little is known about the X chromosome compared to the Y chromosome (see page 100), partly because researchers have been far more interested in how the latter causes male development! None the less, recent work has identified three pieces of the genetic jigsaw on the X chromosome that are vital for ovarian development. Researchers have also discovered a rare 'fragile X syndrome', which is inherited within certain families and may cause premature ovarian failure in some cases by affecting the menopausal body-clock.[15] Here genetic testing could help doctors to warn some young women in time for them to get pregnant or store frozen embryos.

Women are most likely to lack follicles because their supply has been damaged. Ovarian surgery, hysterectomy and cancer treatments can cause the menopause for this reason (see Chapter 8). A less obvious culprit is an ovarian infection, such as mumps oophoritis. However, this is extremely rare and mumps is better known as an illness to be avoided by men because it can cause painful testicular failure.

Ironically ovarian failure is much more likely to be due to a misguided attack by the body's immune system than a case of mumps.

The immune system is designed to tell the difference between body cells and intruders, such as harmful bacteria and viruses. One of the ways it does this is by producing antibodies, which identify and destroy unwelcome cells. Sometimes the process gets confused and produces *auto*-antibodies, which attack body cells ('auto' means 'self'). This happens quite often in women with premature ovarian failure. For example, one study found auto-immunity in 40 per cent of such women compared to 3.6 per cent of similar women without ovarian failure.[16] Auto-antibodies against the thyroid gland were most common (see Monique, below). Premature ovarian failure is also associated with other glandular auto-immune problems, such as Addison's disease, which affects the adrenals.

No one knows what the link between some cases of premature ovarian failure and auto-immunity really means. The link suggests that auto-immunity may be the reason why some women's ovaries, and perhaps other glands, stop working. Yet tests have shown that auto-antibodies can be present without leading to recognizable signs or symptoms. For example, one study found that a group of women with premature ovarian failure had similar previous menstrual patterns, hormone, scan and bone-density results[17] – whether they had auto-antibodies or not. Also, there are few signs of auto-*ovarian* antibodies in such patients[18] (although this may be because researchers haven't found the best way to detect and measure them rather than anything else).[19] It may be that auto-immunity makes follicles unresponsive, but doctors are still trying to clarify whether this is so and if it can be reversed.

Often the reason for a premature menopause is unclear and women are obliged to accept that doctors cannot discover the exact cause in their case or – since most cases of ovarian failure cannot be reversed – that they may not even try.

Hormone Treatment

A woman with premature menopause can feel she has suffered the shock of a major illness and yet find the diagnosis is regarded quite lightly by her doctor, unless she wants fertility treatment. From a gynaecologist's point of view, ovarian failure is simple compared to other conditions they treat, i.e. often little can be done to find the cause, but drugs will replace the missing hormones and no further treatment is required by a specialist. Their attitude may be that it is an early, but otherwise natural, event that has a relatively easy answer in the use of the Pill or HRT (comparatively familiar drugs to patients and therefore thought to be more acceptable). However, this can add up to a set of painful contradictions for women, who often leave the consulting room feeling that their problems haven't been taken seriously.

Usually women with premature ovarian failure are prescribed HRT to treat their menopausal symptoms and reduce the likelihood of later heart disease and osteoporosis, since they have an increased risk of these problems compared to other women their age. They need to take a combined form of HRT to protect the lining of the womb. This treatment will produce regular 'periods' or withdrawal bleeds, which may – or may not – provide a welcome sense of normality.

Sometimes women are prescribed the Pill as hormone replacement because it is contraceptive, whereas HRT is not. This may seem irrelevant, but women with ovarian failure do have an unpredictable chance of pregnancy and not everyone is willing or ready to take this risk. Some women opt for the Pill because it is familiar, easier to explain away and, in the UK, free of prescription charges, unlike HRT (combined HRT can attract a double fee). However, the Pill is not appropriate for long-term use as hormone replacement because it doesn't provide continuous oestrogen (only three weeks in every month), unlike most HRT (see also page 114). Also, some women find it embarrassing or too painful a reminder to be on the Pill, having probably lost their fertility.

Women with premature ovarian failure can feel that their bodies have been 'fast-forwarded', so that they will now age as if they *were* 50 years old. This fear is very understandable. However, women have not skipped 20–30 years of life because of an early menopause. They do have extra risks of problems associated with later life, such as heart disease and osteoporosis, although these risks can be reduced with HRT.

Fertility Treatments

Sometimes doctors check whether drugs will stimulate ovulation in women with premature ovarian failure. For example, a GP may be willing to prescribe drugs such as Clomid (see Diane, below) or a specialist clinic may try various (often somewhat experimental) techniques to get a response from the ovaries. All such attempts require careful monitoring.

Even if a woman cannot produce active follicles or ovulate, she may be able to have a child or complete her family through egg-donation IVF. As its name suggests, this type of 'test-tube baby' treatment involves eggs donated by another woman. The eggs are fertilized by sperm from the patient's partner. Then up to three embryos are introduced into the patient's womb in the hope that one will implant. The procedure is fairly simple, although tricky to get right (see Figure 7.2). If the couple wish, any remaining embryos of suitable quality can be frozen for future attempts. At present, unfertilized eggs cannot be frozen without a high risk of damage and so embryos are stored instead. However, embryos do not always survive thawing and the chances of pregnancy are lower with those that do. None the less, children have been born without harm from frozen embryos.

Some people object to IVF on religious or moral grounds. Usually they are concerned about the status of each embryo because IVF involves producing embryos in a laboratory and some may be discarded or frozen. Egg-donation IVF can lead to further objections because it relies on eggs from another woman. Couples who do not

Figure 7.2 Stages of egg-donation IVF for women who cannot ovulate[20]

- Specialized HRT is used to co-ordinate the patient's cycle with the donor's and make the patient's uterus more receptive.
- Eggs collected from the donor are fertilized with sperm from the patient's partner; embryos won't develop from every egg, although half a dozen may be produced.
- Two to four days later, a maximum of three embryos at the 'four-cell stage' are ushered through the patient's cervix in the hope that one will implant in her womb. This procedure does not require a general anaesthetic.
- Any remaining embryos are frozen (if this is acceptable to those concerned).
- If the patient conceives, hormonal drugs are continued until her body takes over (usually about eight weeks into the pregnancy).
- About 34 per cent of women with ovarian failure will get a positive pregnancy test;[21] even fewer will take a baby home as the general miscarriage rate may be 15 per cent.

N.B. This describes the transfer of 'fresh' embryos; some clinics only transfer frozen embryos. This can depend on the way donors are recruited and tested.

object to this idea on principle may still need to come to terms with the idea of egg donation.

Even if egg-donation IVF is acceptable, it is not an easy or simple choice – physically, emotionally or financially. In the UK there are few NHS infertility clinics and health authorities have different criteria for acceptance, although national guidelines are being developed. Couples able to afford a private clinic find that they must join a long waiting list because of the shortage of egg donors. The shortage is partly because egg donation is a much more demanding experience than sperm donation. Sometimes sisters act as egg donors, although this is not necessarily advisable (see HFEA, page 276). Even when couples reach the top of the waiting list, the chances of failure are high. However, once pregnant, patients with ovarian failure are just as likely to carry a baby as other women.[22]

Although egg-donation IVF is not especially hazardous, it can be very stressful because of the intensive timetabling and the inevitable emotional rollercoaster. There is a lot to consider, so it is worth getting detailed guidance on how to choose a clinic and what to expect when one gets there (see More Help).

Adoption is always put forward as the alternative to fertility treatment. However, this is not an easy option either. Adoption agencies also have long waiting lists (see Diane, below) and they can be very selective about who they will accept as prospective parents. Further information about adoption, fostering and surrogacy is available from relevant organizations (see More Help).

Women's Stories

Andrea

Since starting at 11, I'd always had regular periods and they'd never been particularly heavy or painful. Shortly after my 15th birthday, my periods started coming every two weeks. I went on holiday to Clacton with my cousin and my period was really heavy. I came back on two weeks later. I wasn't particularly concerned, but my Mum told me to go to the doctor, just to check everything was OK.

My GP told me it was nothing to worry about. She said to keep a diary of my periods – how often they came, how heavy, etc. Of course, I never kept the diary, but I never had another period after that August.

I didn't really think anything of it, except 'Oh well, it'll come next month'. To tell the truth, I was pleased not to have the hassle! But around Christmas I started getting hot flushes. They got worse, so I went to my GP who said she needed a blood and urine sample to do some tests. The results didn't show anything, so I had to give more blood. Still nothing was 'abnormal', so I was sent for a scan to check my ovaries. The lady giving it said she thought everything looked in working order.

On April 1, I went back for the scan results – everything was fine. My GP couldn't understand it until she looked back and realized she had not read the results of my second blood test properly, which showed my hormones were unbalanced. She suggested it could be the menopause and said she'd refer me to a gynaecologist. I burst out crying. I don't know why, because I didn't take in a single thing she said. I just felt so numb – like it wasn't really happening to me but to someone else, and I was looking on.

My Mum tried to reassure me, saying my GP was only a general doctor and didn't know everything for definite – she was just speculating.

A month later, I saw the gynaecologist. He said it could be one of two things – I had no eggs, meaning the menopause, or my eggs were not receiving the message to ovulate, which could be corrected. In order to know, he needed more blood samples.

Unfortunately I was revising for my exams and we didn't want them all messed up, so we decided it would be more sensible to get my blood test results after they had finished.

My exams started. I found it really hard to concentrate and my hot flushes were really bad, at least one per hour! I could not stand the suspense – I was going insane not knowing, so I phoned the hospital and asked them to pass on my results.

On Saturday May 24 my Mum told me that my ovaries had failed – I was going through the menopause. I burst into tears. I couldn't believe it was happening. I had already arranged to go out that night; one of my sisters said don't go out if you don't feel up to it. I knew if I stayed in the house I would mope about crying. So I went out and got really drunk – I've read alcohol is good for women with the menopause!!!

I went back to the gynaecologist. He explained about the menopause and said the easiest thing to get rid of hot flushes, to bring my periods and to prevent osteoporosis would be the Pill. I was given Ovysmen and told I would need a bone-density scan in five years' time. The Pill gave me headaches at first, but it has settled down. The only drawback is having to have periods.

The thing that annoyed me was the fact that my hot flushes, etc., could have been sorted out before my exams, instead of four months later. I have lost all confidence in my GP. But the worst of it is that I had the chance to have children, and now that has been taken away from me. I feel robbed and let down. Only my family and friends at work know about my condition. I just can't bring myself to tell my friends – I don't want them to pity me – or think I'm a freak. I feel as if I have let my family down. I will dread it in years to come when I find someone to settle down with – what if I don't, because I can't give them a child?

I work in a fashion shop on a Saturday and I never realized how many babies can actually come in in one day. Everywhere I turn there is a pram or a baby buggy. Whenever I see a young girl with a child, I always think what I wouldn't give to be in her position. You don't realize what you've got until it's gone.

Jayne

As a staff nurse, I realized something was not quite right. My periods, which had always been somewhat erratic, stopped completely. I was 26.

I waited five months before seeking advice from my GP. Over the subsequent months I made many visits to this man. First with constipation, for which he gave me laxatives; secondly with mood swings, forgetfulness and irritability, for which he prescribed anti-depressants. Then I developed what looked like severe acne on my lower body. For this he suggested vitamins. Even with this concoction of medicines, there was no improvement.

A year after my periods had stopped, I was referred to a gynaecologist who carried out blood tests, ultrasound and a magnetic resonance test. The MRI scan indicated that I had a small pituitary adenoma and my care was transferred to an endocrinologist. He explained that the adenoma was not affecting my pituitary gland. However, I was feeling more and more unwell.

Tiredness took on a whole new meaning – I could barely manage a shift and was asleep in bed when not on the ward. 'Acne' covered my thighs, hips and back, and I began to experience tingling in my legs, like spiders creeping up and down my skin. I was emotional, forgetful and then came the hot flushes. Whatever had happened to the girl who approached life with boundless energy and enthusiasm? I really thought I was dying. The signs were all there; however, the menopause seemed a bizarre thought.

Close friends and family saw the change in me. How they put up with me, I'll never know. However, their love and loyalty, coupled with my strong faith, sustained me during those uncertain days and continues to do so.

Two months on I was signed off work with exhaustion, while awaiting blood results. November 15 was a day that changed my life for ever. In the clinic I was sensitively informed that my ovaries had 'packed up' – premature ovarian failure. There appeared to be no logical reason for this. The pituitary was working normally, despite the small tumour.* However, the ovaries were not responding to its messages.

Initially I experienced relief. HRT would replace the severely depleted oestrogen in my body; I could return to work and some normality. I wasn't dying. The relief, however, was short-lived. These feelings were replaced by anger and disbelief. I felt a freak, not normal.

Four months after starting Mercilon, I returned to work part-time. When I started to have severe headaches, my medication was changed to Microgynon 30.

I was single and without children, but had not ruled out getting married and having a family. I loved children (I had specialized in paediatrics) and now the ability to have my own had been snatched

* Note: Benign pituitary tumours are quite common so this was coincidental and not causing Jayne's early menopause.

from me. Who would want me like this? The whole idea of relationships scared me; how could I ever tell anyone? I didn't want to consider it.

That Christmas, just after I was diagnosed, I met a bloke through mutual friends. We became good friends. I really thought he knew; he never asked why I was off work, so I assumed someone had told him. After about a year we became romantically involved. I immediately realized that he had no idea. I panicked and told him. It was horrendous and I probably didn't handle the situation very well. Nothing could have prepared me for his reaction, it was so hurtful. He treated me completely differently, but I was the same girl. He mumbled, 'Does that mean you can't have children?', followed by, 'I must go home.' Then he left and that was the end, although he phoned later to say that he couldn't cope. So my fears had been realized – I'd been dumped because I wasn't a proper woman.

After this rejection, I was forced to confront how I felt about the illness and its bearing on my life. Prior to that I had just busied myself. On reflection, I equate it to a bereavement – part of me had died and I was passing through the grieving process described in my nurse training: denial, anger, bargaining, depression, acceptance. Oh yes, acceptance – that's a tough one – will I truly reach that stage?

My faith, friends and family were steadfast in this latest setback on the road to acceptance. My oestrogen levels were dropping again, which didn't help. Some of my symptoms returned, especially during the week off medication. My HRT was changed to Tridestra, which contains a different oestrogen and dose, taken in a three-monthly cycle. I seem much better on this drug, hopefully this is the right one.

In all honesty, some days still appear very black. Lots of my friends have babies and at times I find it really difficult. The fact that the ovaries kick-start in 5 per cent of cases and the possibility of egg-donation IVF mean that having a family is not out of the question, although premature menopause is a major hurdle when it comes to relationships. The first reaction I encountered was clumsy, insensitive and extremely distressing. However, the second was more favourable.

This time it didn't matter at all. He wasn't the one for me, but he did restore my faith in men a bit. I still can't say when or how to break the news, but you just have to live and learn. Living through a premature menopause is a horrific experience and it affects every aspect of your life. In the meantime I pray daily that I am granted the courage, fortitude and ability to carry on with life as positively as I can.

Julia

Six years ago, I collapsed at work and was found to be so anaemic I needed a blood transfusion. I had a tennis-ball-sized fibroid and underwent major surgery. I was told I was lucky to have avoided a hysterectomy. I was 31.

During the following year I began feeling unwell, including panic attacks and palpitations. Investigations with a cardiologist proved normal, but my odd symptoms continued and I began to suffer flushes, sweating and other menopausal symptoms. My periods had been irregular since my op, with spotting sometimes for several weeks. I had a D&C, but no cause was found. Although I didn't feel well, there seemed to be no explanation. A new GP checked my hormones and eventually confirmed that I was menopausal.

I was shocked and distressed. I was still young enough to have hopes of marriage and children. I felt angry, blaming the surgeon. I also felt I had been through so much to save my womb, only to find it was useless anyway.

A chromosome analysis found that 6 per cent of the cells lacked an X chromosome. The consultant said this could be a mosaic of Turner syndrome [see page 108], but would not commit himself because I had normal ovaries and had started menstruating at 12 with textbook periods from ages 15 to 25.

I have decided that the surgery was probably not to blame, although there is still a tiny doubt in my mind. I have been given very little information and what I have been told has at times been contradictory and confusing. I have never once been asked how I feel. My GP said I was being 'too introspective' when I wished to find out more, and more or less told me to take the HRT she was offering and go away and forget about it.

Initially I was put on Prempak-C 0.625 mg and then 1.25 mg, which I took for a year. Although it helped some symptoms (flushing and sweating, joint pains and lack of energy), I felt depressed, at times crying helplessly for no reason. Other side-effects included heartburn and very painful periods. I was then advised by my consultant to try the Pill, but I didn't get on with that too well either.

I haven't taken any treatment for the last five months. I am now 37 and my consultant says that if I really don't want HRT, I will have to work harder to protect my bones and circulation by exercising more and increasing my calcium intake. My mother has osteoporosis and there is a family history of circulatory problems, so these are additional risks. I am waiting for a bone scan, which should help me decide. I would like to investigate natural remedies.

It is perhaps an exaggeration to say this has blighted my life, but I do feel this sometimes. I suppose I have always been the retiring type, but I have lost a lot of confidence and my work prospects and social life have also suffered. I am not in a relationship and do not expect to have children, but still feel sad about this, particularly when I see friends and relatives in their late thirties or even early forties conceiving without apparent difficulty. The late thirties can be a broody time for any childless woman without the added stress of coping with the menopause and HRT. As an only child, I also feel I have let my mother down by not giving her grandchildren.

The menopause is such a taboo subject and so difficult to discuss. It definitely makes it worse if you can't talk about your situation or explain why you're depressed or, perhaps, behaving oddly. For me, one of the worst aspects is the isolation. I have wondered how much of what I was going through was caused by the hormones or really psychological. Sometimes it felt like I was going quietly mad.

I am very aware that the menopause is a natural process and I've felt ashamed that I couldn't cope with something that isn't a problem for other people. I feel guilty too as I know there are much worse things that can happen. Early menopause is, after all, not life threatening.

In the past few months I have at last come to terms with having an early menopause. I feel calmer and less resentful, but I still find it difficult to deal with what has happened. I will probably go back on HRT, but am not sure I want to take it for 15–20 years, as my GP initially advised. I hope to get some of my confidence back and to sort out my life, but I can't really expect HRT to do this for me. I know it can't work miracles.

Pippa

I had one natural period, aged 14. Then I went on the Pill and had withdrawal bleeds as one does with oral contraceptives. It never occurred to me that something might be amiss until I came off the Pill at 24 and ceased bleeding altogether. My GP said it was probably because I'd taken the Pill for so long, and my natural cycle would reinstate itself all in good time.

Two years later I was referred to a gynaecologist who conducted various tests, ultrasound scans, etc. He finally diagnosed premature ovarian failure, although he was unable to tell me the cause. I remember only too well: it was my 26th birthday when he said I would never be able to have my own children, except possibly by egg donation.

I have subsequently married, very happily, but unfortunately my husband and I are not in a financial position to try for IVF. My husband has a grown-up son by his first marriage, so I don't think he is too worried. But I would have liked to have a baby of my own. However, it was not to be and, at 38, I have resigned myself.

I have been on HRT for over 10 years now, trying both patches and tablets in various forms, e.g. Prempak-C, Trisequens and Kliofem. Kliofem was the best, symptom-wise, except for loss of libido, which caused a few problems with my husband. He does his best to understand the situation, but it's not easy for either of us.

Recently I began Evorel patches combined with Micronor tablets, so that I get a monthly withdrawal bleed. I was initially on 50 mg patches but this was increased to 75 mg to try and counteract my symptoms, i.e. vaginal dryness, loss of libido, etc., etc.!

Long-term, I am worried about the effects of HRT, but my current GP doesn't seem to think it is an important subject for discussion! I also worry about the increased risk of breast cancer, but nobody will refer me for a mammogram, which I feel would help put my mind at rest, if nothing else [see pages 97–8]. However, I feel better on my new HRT and have managed to lose weight, which I am delighted about. I feel that I must persevere with the treatment and accept that it is an ongoing thing.

Since discovering the Premature Menopause Support Group I feel some people have sympathy for me – it's really great to meet women with the same troubles. I don't think any 'ordinary' woman would have any idea what it is like to go through all this with little support from the medics.

Antonia

I always wanted a family and waited until the time seemed right. At last, it seemed like life was beginning: I was 35, in a relationship and we both wanted children very much.

Months passed, but as my partner travelled on business a lot I made excuses and waited. After 18 months, I went to the fertility clinic. Blood was taken, past history discussed and a week later the first result showed raised FSH level. This, I was told, was the first sign of menopause, but could be a laboratory blip and must be repeated. After the second test I received a call to attend the clinic urgently, which I did, only to be told quite bluntly that I had premature ovarian failure; it would be a miracle for me to conceive and the only hope of having a child was by egg donation.

To say I was stunned doesn't begin to describe my feelings. I went home in a daze, convinced my partner would no longer want me. To my relief, I received his full support, but the implications of my diagnosis were eating away at the back of my mind. Menopause books were of no use as all they told me was that by now my children would have left home and I would be thinking of retirement! Nothing could have been further from the truth.

I felt very alone with no one I could speak to about how I felt. For years the trend has been for couples to start their families late and I had no idea that premature ovarian failure affected as many as 1 per cent of women. I can remember being taught the facts of life by people trying to protect young girls by saying that 'it only takes once', and here I was after months of trying and it was all over before I had started.

We began the long haul of choosing a private clinic, but being spoilt for choice in London was actually a blessing. We chose the clinic closest to work and I was amazed to be offered a one-off attempt at GIFT. The medical team had had some success treating women with sub-optimal results and felt strongly that every woman should have one chance of conception with her own eggs. The cost was high and we were counselled that it had a very slim chance of success, but at least we would have tried.

I was put on maximum-dose IVF drugs, but my first scan showed no response and although I continued for a few days, I never did produce any eggs. The staff were very supportive and offered counselling, but in some ways I was more depressed than the first time. As much as you tell yourself you don't expect good news, you don't realize how high your hopes were until they are dashed.

Although we are on a waiting list for an egg donor, we are currently taking a break as it can make you feel you have no control over anything and it all becomes very stressful. In the meantime, I am focusing on my mental and physical health. I'm not on HRT just now and don't get many hot flushes, although I often feel lethargic. All this has taken a toll and sometimes I don't know what's being caused by depression and what's being caused by the menopause. Mentally I'm facing life head-on and thinking what path to take if all fertility attempts fail or we decide the techniques available aren't appropriate. The thought of spending all our waking time obsessing about achieving pregnancy horrifies us and we need time off the 'conveyor belt' to think things through.

My diagnosis filled a lot of gaps about the last few years. Lots of symptoms, meaningless on their own, gradually made sense: the sudden weight gain after years of being the same size regardless of what I ate, waking up dripping in sweat during the night and a pervading sense of lethargy when before I was out every night and had a reputation for never sitting still. It is a relief to have a diagnosis, but losing my fertility feels as if something has died. I regret leaving it so long before asking for help and advise all my friends to get checked out as soon as possible. When I was phoning clinics for their prospectus, they would comment on how young I was. I had to explain that when you've been told you're menopausal you feel anything but young!

Monique

Five years ago, I conceived very easily and gave birth to a healthy baby boy. I was 33. My periods were quite regular after I stopped breastfeeding, but when James was a year old, I decided to go on a diet to lose some post-pregnancy weight. After a short time my periods stopped, which I put down to losing weight. They started again, somewhat erratically, after I reached my target. However, they were late and every month I thought I was pregnant, only to have negative test after negative test. It was a difficult time. Then they stopped completely.

I waited for a couple of months (and a few more pregnancy tests) before going to my doctor. He thought I might have a blighted ovum, but a scan showed no signs of this. The ultrasonographer said my ovaries appeared to be shut down. My GP arranged a blood test and, when it showed high FSH and LH, he said I'd had a premature menopause.

At first I was shocked, but not unduly concerned. I had never heard of this and assumed that with a course of hormones, my body would sort itself out. I soon found out that it was irreversible. I was devastated as we badly wanted to complete our family. My doctor said our only hope was egg donation. He also mentioned I would have to spend 15 or so years taking HRT to protect me from osteoporosis and heart disease.

As my main focus was to have a baby, we went on to a waiting list for a donor. My younger sister also offered to donate eggs. We spent quite a long time deciding what to do, how we felt, how to fund it and so on. Eventually, in September last year, we embarked on the egg-donation treadmill with my sister. Once we started, the whole process was quite quick and by Christmas we knew the egg collection would be at the end of January. I took my first dose of Cyclo-Progynova as part of the fertility treatment.

The egg collection went extremely well. My sister produced 24 eggs! My husband felt quite daunted! How many would he be able to fertilize? Nineteen were fertilized, of which three were transferred to my womb two days later. The attempt failed. Twelve embryos were frozen and in April we tried again. Again, none survived.

Since then I have been unable to try again. The first failure was particularly painful, as my sister and I lost our father on Christmas Day. I felt, quite irrationally, that as God had taken away my father, He would give me a baby instead. Of course, things do not work out that neatly in real life. The second failure was also very hard, and I felt I could not try again until I had redressed the balance of my life. James is my first concern: he exists now and needs me now and I cannot spend his precious childhood chasing the dream of a child that may never exist.

At the moment we still have six frozen embryos. I am much happier now than I was. James is a delightful, energetic little boy who is a constant source of pleasure (and exhaustion!). I have been taking Cyclo-Progynova as HRT and feel much better for it. My two complaints are putting on weight and that my libido is not quite what it was. I am also doing what I can to help my body: I manage a swim twice a week, do as much walking as I can and take various vitamin and mineral supplements.

We are about to embark on another attempt at having our elusive second child. Once I have either become pregnant or decided to accept the cards life has dealt me, I will continue to take HRT. I shall, however, look for another type that enables me (hopefully) to lose that little bit of weight and, more importantly, revives my flagging sexual desire.

I do not like the idea of taking HRT long-term, but I see, and feel, its benefits and as I have a young child, I want to stay alive and in good health to look after him. My symptoms have virtually disappeared and I no longer wake in the night drenched in sweat.

Two years after I was diagnosed with premature menopause I sometimes feel bitter. But I am one of the lucky ones: I know why it happened (I had Hashimoto's thyroiditis at 17 and have been on thyroxine ever since) and I have a much-loved child. Also, I am lucky enough to afford egg donation and blessed that my sister had the generosity to donate eggs.

Diane

Three years ago, aged 36, I was diagnosed as post-menopausal. Looking back, the signs had been evident for several years and now I think we are very lucky to have a child at all. My son was born when I was 33.

Since starting at 11, my periods were always somewhat erratic and painful. After I got married at 30, I no longer knew how heavy or long they would be. My GP was not sympathetic and even suggested that I really wanted her to stop my periods altogether – rather ironic now. However, she sent me to a gynaecologist, whose advice was to start a family.

About twelve months later, I became pregnant without any effort (or so it seemed). I felt wonderful throughout my pregnancy. I breastfed and my periods started almost six months after James's birth.

When James was a year old, I missed two periods and developed night sweats. I thought I was pregnant, but a test proved negative. My GP advised a holiday, which we were already going on, and said to come back if necessary. My period started on holiday.

The following 18 months were very stressful. We sold our house, lived with family for a year and there were management changes at work. My periods became totally unpredictable, which I put down to stress. Then I went two months without a period and started hot flushes. A pregnancy test was negative. My new GP sent me for blood tests, which indicated I'd had the menopause.

My new GP was very supportive. He sent me for monthly tests in case this was a temporary blip in my system. I was given Clomid to kick-start my ovaries, but with no success. Initially we could not accept that nothing could be done, so we sought a second and third opinion. They just said I must go on HRT and egg donation was my only option. They did not appear to appreciate how devastating this was to someone my age.

My feelings went from disbelief to anger to sadness and despair. My life and future had just been taken away from me. I felt guilty about not giving my son a brother or sister and my husband the other children he had always wanted. This was made worse because *I* had delayed having a second child 'until later' when we were settled. Now it was too late. I needed someone to talk and cry with, someone who understood the loss, mourning and total desolation. My husband's sense of loss was as great, but mine involved another dimension. Everyday I waited for a sign that it might be a mistake, then I'd have another hot flush and realize it was for real.

Overnight I felt I had become an old woman. My body had let me down and I no longer understood it. I was always very tired, my sex drive was/is non-existent. I was determined to cope without HRT – I don't want to be taking anything for 20 years or so. My mother had deep vein thrombosis twice, initially due to hormone treatment. No one has explained to me why taking hormones for contraception has greater risks than taking them as replacement therapy [see pages 213–14]. Do I or don't I take HRT????

Some days I have no energy and my family suffers as a result. When I feel like this, I admit defeat and decide to ask for HRT. Next day I have loads of energy, so I leave it. Then I go mad not knowing how long this energy will last. Is this going to be the pattern of life from now on?

I am very conscious of my health risks and know I have a duty to my son and husband. Initially I saw a nutritionist and started taking herbal and vitamin supplements, but I gave up because the cost did not justify my results. For the last nine months I have taken 1000 mg of starflower oil per day, which has helped, especially the migraines I was having. Recently my GP prescribed calcium supplements in the lemon powders to drink once a day. I have also been using HRT vaginal cream.

I've felt very angry that doctors appear to give no consideration to this problem. More and more women are going to be affected as they delay starting a family. If the numerous doctors I had seen with 'period problems' had explored my family history, perhaps I would have been advised to have children earlier. My mother had her menopause when she was 40-ish. My slightly older sister has begun experiencing hot flushes, erratic periods, etc.

I felt that as the one woman per year with this problem seen by the gynaecologist, I was expected to go away and get on with my life. I do know, as one doctor suggested, that compared to many younger women in my position, I am very lucky to have a child. But this is not how we planned our life. It breaks my heart to see my son sitting on his swing in the garden all by himself. And it is still very painful seeing others with babies, especially friends who had their first child when I had James and now have their second and third.

Two years ago we decided to pursue the lengthy process of adoption. This April, we were approved, but our son is now six and we feel it may soon be too late for us. Hopefully women in the future need not run out of time.

Susan

I had my first period aged 12. A second followed and then no more. Early menopause was not diagnosed until I was 19 and a laparotomy revealed shrunken ovaries and 'infantile' pelvic organs.

What had happened? My kindly gynaecologist couldn't say. It was just one of those things. Outwardly I took it on the chin; inside, my damaged self-confidence would affect me in many ways over the next few years.

Firstly, there was the question of hormone replacement. With my low oestrogen and high FSH levels, the consultant insisted on redressing the balance. What would happen if I failed to take my pills, I asked? Not a great deal in the short term, he replied. Long-term, possibly osteoporosis and heart disease.

I was warned to expect some discomfort initially. A little breast tenderness perhaps, some water retention. Mood swings or nausea might appear, but the situation would stabilize after three months. With these expectations, I went back to college. Within weeks my clothes became tighter. Tender breasts and black mood swings, coupled with unbelievable tension, became the order of the day.

I finally took unauthorized leave from HRT, rapidly losing the weight I'd accumulated. Ironically I'd had no menopausal symptoms in the six period-free years of my so-called adolescence. Then I'd gone on HRT and when I came off it I found out what all the fuss was about!* The innocuous appearance of those tiny pills belied their real power. I hadn't realized they could literally 'change' a person.

Thus began my uneasy relationship with HRT. Everything I read pointed to the need to monitor blood pressure and reassess the value of each preparation. Instead I was left to my own devices and my (very) uncomfortable side-effects dismissed, albeit politely, as neurotic whinges. This was coupled with an overwhelming need to be seen to be coping; after all, the condition wasn't life threatening, was it? I should count myself lucky to have something that was at least invisible and did not require regular hospitalization.

It was the very invisibility of premature menopause that caused the problems. Those close to me took the doctor's view that, apart from infertility, I was a 'perfectly normal young woman'. There was no breakdown, no real illness in evidence. Just the slow chipping away at my self-image. The self-confidence that had steadily eroded during my teens because I did not 'manage' to keep having periods

---

* It seems that women can only get hot flushes when their bodies have been sensitized by sufficient oestrogen, usually at puberty. Susan was sensitized by her HRT instead and therefore suffered hot flushes when she stopped taking it.

also prevented me from choosing a path in life and I left college directionless and lacking identity.

The weight problem returned when I started HRT again, changing the person I saw in the mirror (even after all these years, I feel it's not me). Without medical support and unable to make sense of what was happening, I became withdrawn. Having seen me diagnosed as a bubbly 19-year-old, close family did not understand that this new me was related to my medical condition. Though I was plainly unwell for someone my age, no one knew enough at that time to recognize why and offer support. The doctor, everyone, put the weight gain down to 'overeating'.

I was lucky to have a partner; someone unfailingly supportive and understanding. When we met at college, I'd never had a date. My upbringing and lack of periods had combined to persuade me that I would be abnormal in personal relationships too, and sexuality was something I had no right to because of my medical condition. On the outside I was outgoing, even flamboyant, yet I shied away from boys, afraid of initiating something that would expose me as a physical 'fraud'. I don't exactly understand what I was afraid of. I only know that, on some level, I'd read enough about the menopause to feel I had not developed adequately for physical relations. When I met Keith I found someone determined to pursue me, who found me very physically attractive and told me so. I let him believe the packs of HRT were contraceptives and eventually, after many months of platonic relationship, I took the plunge!

It was almost a shock to find that, to him, I was a normal, full-blooded 20-year-old. I had half expected confirmation of my freak-ishness. After some months I came clean about the little pills. I explained that I didn't need contraception and my ovaries didn't work. It was all very low-key. The next surprise was that it made no difference at all.

At 24 we married. We both knew children were not an option and it was never an issue for Keith. At this stage I didn't experience any anxiety over my infertility. I was more concerned with how to look after my hormonally depleted body. When friends started having children, I shared their joy. Only one friendship dissolved because, as I saw it, she was careless with words. Continuous tactlessness, rather than isolated incidents, can be quite soul-destroying! One thing I've always been clear about, even at my lowest ebb, is that fertility is not linked to one's value as a human being.

When I finally started teaching, the physical demands were very difficult. Despite being on Progynova by now, I regularly experienced hot flushes. Once home I crashed on the sofa, unable to move. The GP would not accept a connection with my medical condition. I saw a gynaecologist who was far more interested in my infertility than my symptoms and delivered a mini-lecture on people who 'wait too long before starting a family'. Having accepted my infertility as irreversible, I found this unhelpful.

He agreed to let me try an implant. This was slightly more useful than the pills. I was thrilled when I continued to have a cyclical period after the implant's supposed six-month duration and without taking progesterone [see page 231]. This blip caused much optimism and my gynaecologist said I was 'on the mend' and he wouldn't be surprised if I got pregnant. I was on cloud nine!

Dashed hopes and infertility treatment followed. Hormones, injections, pills, scans, visits. It felt exciting and purposeful despite the discomforts. I was honestly more thrilled with the notion of normal periods and not relying on HRT than the thought of my 'abstract' baby, as I'd virtually grown up knowing I couldn't have children. That the ovaries might still do their work after eight years or so seemed impossibly exciting because my 'withdrawal bleeds' had never felt real (though I liked having sanipads or tampons in my drawer like every other girl). Needless to say, I was not one of the lucky few who return to normal function.

Back on HRT, the effects of Prempak-C were quite vicious. I had lost a great deal of excess weight after my implant. Now it was piling on again. My breasts were sore, again I was lethargic with severe mood swings, which left me feeling detached from my surroundings. The consultant was adamant that I must continue Prempak-C for the effect to settle down. He dismissed the weight gain.

When I turned 30, I looked back with mounting anger and helplessness. Apparently little had been learned about premature menopause since my diagnosis. The sense of being unique was compounded by a certain lack of interest. I'd imagined that a rare condition would at least provoke interest in my case, a desire to learn more. All the information I received on HRT was about older women and the natural menopause. If no one was listening to me, how could my treatment be appropriate? Were there others out there? Were they being heard? I felt isolated and overlooked by medical wisdom, having spent a decade without a positive way of managing what is basically a glandular condition before it becomes an infertility issue. I was confused, despondent and unwell, having sampled a veritable cocktail of HRT preparations.

It was only through a chance remark, 'Ever thought about IVF with donated eggs?', that I resolved the question of involuntary childlessness. As a very young woman, I had dismissed childbirth as a fearsome, mildly distasteful thing to be avoided. Children I loved and generally got on with. When I realized that I too could join the club of motherhood, I had to re-evaluate my expectations. Firstly, how would I cope with the physical demands and, secondly, was it right to pursue treatment with donated eggs?

The second question was easier to deal with. My body had let me down by not producing eggs. Just one little egg cell – that's all I needed to redress the awful trick Nature had played on me. Oh yes, and plenty of hormones to 'fool' my body into thinking it was pregnant. I still look upon egg-donation IVF as a complex and particularly altruistic form of organ donation. I say 'altruistic' because it is offered actively by donors to help women like myself. It is complex because it involves genetic material and more emotive than sperm donation because it involves mothers, the starting point of all creation.

I became pregnant at our first attempt at IVF. I couldn't believe it, conditioned as I was to expect disappointment. It was such a shock, after believing for so long that 'you couldn't put a baby in there' (as a GP had said to me). The pregnancy made me very tired and I became paranoid about resting. I was injected with Gestone daily for the first 14 weeks, tailing off at 16 weeks. It was nerve-racking, like having your water-wings pulled off and being expected to swim when there's no guarantee that you can!

My baby boy arrived a few weeks early and the mixture of uncontrollable joy, relief at having delivered him safely and disbelief at being a mother almost proved too much! Considering the amount of technology involved in his conception, I was given little information afterwards. I didn't know how quickly to go back on HRT, for instance. In the absence of any precise data, the obstetrician indicated, in the nicest possible way, that this was a matter of personal choice. I was, and still am, very disappointed that HRT can be prescribed in situations that are outside the research available. I was expected to take responsibility for my well-being and that of my newborn, something I would prefer to do when in full possession of the facts!*

With little warning of what was to come, the aftermath was a physical and mental shock. I lost a great deal of blood in the month after giving birth. In the first year, I had backache from the difficult epidural and terrible joint pains; stiffness that made mundane tasks such as pushing a supermarket trolley painful. Tiredness from looking after my beloved but highly strung little one made me chronically unwell. Another IVF attempt using the remaining frozen embryos ended in miscarriage. A year of ill health followed and I continued to pile on weight.

I decided to consider the very-low-fat diets I had previously scorned. A slimming club helped me shed 14 lb and adopting a few dietary principles did the same again. Cutting out caffeine and dairy produce and taking supplements boosted my almost non-existent energy levels. I now look upon vegetables as medicine, something to be chosen carefully and cooked to get maximum nutritional benefit.

* Unfortunately the necessary studies are unlikely to be done given the few women in this position and the ethics of 'experimenting' with them (see Chapter 9) Breastfeeding is a contraindication to HRT.

I am facing the future with renewed optimism. I am determined that today's young girls with premature menopause should have an easier ride. Then again, I've had an easier ride than others. My advice is to make friends with a gynaecologist and stay in touch with developments.

8

SURGICAL AND MEDICAL MENOPAUSE

*'I'd had time to think and talk to my husband, time to prepare,
or so I thought. But nothing could have prepared me for the
trauma. I had a whole range of feelings and thoughts. Those of
anger, grief and emptiness and that old chestnut, "why me?"'*

TERESA

If younger women's ovaries are removed, they will go through an
immediate 'surgical' menopause and are more likely to suffer osteoporosis and heart disease in later years. HRT can be prescribed to
prevent symptoms and reduce the extra risks, but women could need
prescriptions for decades and the implications are unclear. Usually
women face this decision knowingly and in consultation with their
doctor. However, some women have faced it unknowingly, even
unnecessarily.

Surgery isn't the only medical intervention that can lead to an early
menopause. Radiotherapy and chemotherapy can harm the store of
egg follicles in the ovaries, a store that cannot be renewed by the
body. This means that younger women with cancer may have to cope
with infertility, lack of sex hormones and a 'medical' menopause as
a side-effect of their treatment (although sometimes the ovaries can
recover).

This chapter begins by looking at why doctors advise removing
the ovaries, often during a hysterectomy, and whether this is always
justified. It describes what happens during a surgical menopause and
then goes on to explain how cancer therapies can cause a medical
menopause. Women who have been through this type of menopause
talk about their experiences of coping with illness and the conse-

quences of their treatment. This includes women diagnosed with problems such as recurrent cysts, endometriosis, ovarian cancer, Hodgkin's disease and leukaemia.

Why Women Lose Their Ovaries

Women suspected of having ovarian problems are often referred for an ultrasound scan, which can reveal whether their ovaries are enlarged and, if so, in what way. The scan may show one or more large fluid-filled cysts. Alternatively the surface of the ovary may be bubbled with many small cysts. Occasionally the scan reveals a solid ovarian mass. One or both ovaries may be affected.

Ovarian cysts are common and can occur for all sorts of reasons. In fact, there are over 200 kinds and textbooks delight in listing their strange characteristics, such as the teeth and hair found in 'dermoid' cysts (because of an early mix-up in cell programming). However, most cysts are simply accidents during ovulation. For example, an ovarian follicle will grow into a follicular cyst if it doesn't burst to release its egg, although usually the body reabsorbs the cyst within a cycle or two. A more serious cyst can occur if the follicle bursts as expected, but things go awry when the remaining sac becomes a corpus luteum. Often a small amount of blood is lost when the follicle bursts, but extra bleeding can mean that the sac becomes a dark corpus luteum cyst.

Ovarian cysts can reach the size of oranges or more, often without symptoms. Yet even a smaller cyst can cause problems if it twists the walnut-sized ovary out of position. Twisting can reduce the chances of pregnancy and may block or tear the ovary's blood supply. If bleeding occurs, matters worsen. Eventually the ovary may be squashed thin or pulled apart by the expanding surface of the cyst. This can happen without causing more than a dull ache, occasional mid-cycle pain or blood spotting. But if the cyst ruptures, it will cause severe pain (see Jane, Chapter 1) and often requires emergency surgery (see Clair, below).

Most cysts are caught before they burst. As a general rule, gynae-cologists will operate if an ovarian cyst is 5 cm or more with the aim of preserving fertility in younger women by leaving one or both ovaries or part of an ovary. However, complete removal (oophorectomy) may be advised if cysts are a recurring problem (see Teresa, below).

Sometimes a scan shows ovaries enlarged by many tiny cysts rather than one or two sizeable ones. In polycystic ovarian syndrome (PCOS), the ovaries have a layer of tiny bubbles (no more than 0.5 cm) below the surface and ovulation is disrupted. PCOS is usually treated hormonally, although oophorectomy may be suggested in severe cases.

Occasionally a scan will show a solid ovarian mass rather than a fluid-filled cyst. A solid growth is more likely to be malignant, but ovarian cancer can be difficult to diagnose – even during surgery. Sometimes the surgeon can only reach a conclusion by removing an ovary and waiting, in the middle of the operation, while lab staff prepare a frozen section (slice) and examine it microscopically. If they find suspicious cells, the other ovary will be removed (in most cases). This decision may have to be made without consulting the patient (see Lynnette, below).

A scan can help to diagnose ovarian disorders, but sometimes the problem is not the ovaries themselves, but the oestrogen they release as part of the menstrual cycle. That is, the ovaries may be healthy, but the oestrogen they release can contribute to disease elsewhere in the body. In this case, doctors may advise removing *healthy* ovaries. For example, breast cancer depends on oestrogen and so younger women with breast cancer may have their ovaries removed as part of their treatment, although anti-oestrogen drug treatment is more likely now.[1] Oophorectomy is still advised in severe cases of endo-metriosis, a *benign* disorder in which misplaced patches of tissue like the lining of the womb 'grow' and 'bleed' in response to oestrogen. Usually this problem is treated with drugs and/or less drastic surgery initially, but doctors can recommend removing the ovaries as a last resort (this can also be advised if endometriosis has caused large 'chocolate' cysts on the ovaries).

If women are suffering one of the complaints described above, then it is possible to see why removing the ovaries could help and women may welcome the offer. But doctors can suggest oophorectomy at the same time as hysterectomy for a problem like fibroids or heavy bleeding, even though the ovaries are healthy and the problem could be solved by removing the uterus alone (or, increasingly, by more limited surgery or drug treatments). This advice is more difficult to understand and is controversial, particularly for younger women.

Removing Healthy Ovaries – for Whose Sake?

Every year an estimated 90,000 British women have a hysterectomy.[2] Fourteen per cent have their ovaries taken out at the same time.[3] In the USA almost half the women who have a hysterectomy leave hospital without their ovaries.[4]

Many doctors are willing to remove healthy ovaries during hysterectomy 'just in case'. Usually this means 'just in case of ovarian cancer'. Concern about ovarian cancer arises for two reasons. Firstly, it tends to cause symptoms only in its late stages, when it is difficult to treat. Secondly, at present, there is no screening test for ovarian cancer,* like the smear test for cervical cancer. Therefore the only way doctors can prevent ovarian cancer is to take out healthy ovaries whenever they have the 'opportunity' in the hope of removing a pair from a woman who would have developed ovarian cancer otherwise.

Two British doctors have tried to calculate the actual chances of preventing ovarian cancer in this way.[5] Ovarian cancer is rare compared to breast cancer, but more women die of it each year than from cervical cancer. The risk of developing ovarian cancer depends on family history and age: it is greater if a close relative has had the disease, but reduces for all women after their mid-fifties.[6] Using this

---

* Researchers are investigating screening for women with a strong family history of ovarian cancer, but at present the merits are debatable since imprecise testing could do more harm than good.

type of information, the doctors concluded that a surgeon would have to remove 60–120 pairs of healthy-looking ovaries to have a good chance of preventing 1 case of ovarian cancer in a woman at low risk.

This statistic can be reassuring or alarming. Women with ovarian cancer or those who have lost a relative or friend may feel it is worth removing 60–120 pairs of healthy ovaries without knowing who will benefit by not getting such a devastating disease. Judging by one British survey, many gynaecologists would agree with them: 85 per cent would remove healthy ovaries in post-menopausal women.[7] Others find this practice shocking and are campaigning against routine removal (particularly in the USA).[8] They argue that few other healthy organs are removed 'just in case', in women or men, and little is known about the role of ovarian substances in later life.

Some are also concerned about younger women who face a surgical menopause if their ovaries are removed and who become at greater risk of heart disease and osteoporosis: far more likely threats to their health than ovarian cancer. For example, younger women's risk of heart disease doubles when they lose their hormones and their life expectancy may be reduced by at least five years. Many doctors will argue that these extra risks can be reversed by taking HRT, but, in reality, women often abandon long-term treatment without realizing the implications. This recognition has led some doctors to question whether removing healthy ovaries can be justified in younger women at low risk of ovarian cancer.[9]

Current UK estimates suggest that gynaecologists face the question of whether to advise oophorectomy in younger women surprisingly frequently: 1 in 50 British women will have a hysterectomy before age 35 and 1 in 20 before age 40.[10] Of course, some of these patients will have unhealthy ovaries, which simplifies the decision. These figures do not suggest how many patients will have an oophorectomy during their surgery and, if so, for what reasons, but data from elsewhere indicates that most British gynaecologists are still hesitant about routine oophorectomy in pre-menopausal women: only 24 per cent would remove healthy ovaries in 45–49-year-olds (the youngest group mentioned), even though it could be argued that these women are approaching the average menopause age and will have completed any plans for a family.[11] None the less, 24 per cent is a quarter of the profession and their advice will affect a lot of women.

Ironically research suggests that women who *keep* their ovaries during hysterectomy may also have an early menopause. One follow-up study found that after hysterectomy the ovaries can stop working as much as four years earlier than expected.[12] It is impossible to tell how many women in this study would have had an earlier menopause anyway (i.e. without surgery and perhaps due to their health problem), but the findings suggest that hysterectomy can affect the ovaries. This may be because of damage or restriction of their blood supply (which may be unavoidable during such surgery). These results could provide another reason for removing healthy ovaries during hysterectomy 'just in case' – although they are also an argument for asking whether major surgery is the best way forward.

Whatever advice they receive, women need the chance to understand what is being suggested and its implications. However, gynaecologists do not always provide this care. Indeed, a few doctors have removed patients' healthy ovaries during hysterectomy without their signed consent and been subsequently disciplined or struck off when the women concerned sought legal action.[13]

Surgical Menopause

If a woman has her ovaries removed before the natural menopause, she will go through a surgical menopause, often within days. This type of menopause has a reputation for dramatic hot flushes and night sweats, although women's actual experiences vary. For example, a small study of 100 women who'd had a surgical menopause found that insomnia, presumably due to night sweats, was a more frequent problem (48 per cent) than hot flushes (28 per cent).[14] Aches, pains and headaches were also common. Nevertheless, 34 per cent of women had no symptoms at all.

No one knows why symptoms can be so much worse during a

surgical menopause, but the sudden loss of hormones appears to be, quite literally, a 'shock to the system'. During the natural and premature menopause, the pituitary gland responds to the declining number of egg follicles by producing extra FSH in an effort to kick-start the ovaries and continue the menstrual cycle. When the ovaries are removed, it produces even more FSH in a similar attempt. This surge of FSH seems a likely explanation for the severe symptoms, but research suggests that they are triggered by falling oestrogen instead. As explained in Chapter 3, hot flushes are thought to occur when intermittent falls in oestrogen levels disrupt the hypothalamus in the brain. This, in turn, upsets the nearby thermoregulatory centre, which governs body temperature. So the rapid fall in oestrogen levels after oophorectomy may be responsible for the extreme symptoms. Heavier women can have an easier surgical menopause and this may be because they make oestrone in their body fat, which reduces the sudden fall.

Women can develop other problems, such as vaginal dryness. In the small study mentioned above, 38 per cent of the women complained of painful sex (dyspareunia) and 46 per cent reported loss of libido. Vaginal dryness is due to lack of oestrogen and can be a turn-off at the best of times, but researchers have suggested that oophorectomy may lower sex drive *directly* by reducing the supply of androgen hormones. Both testosterone and androstenedione fall by 50 per cent after removal of the ovaries and this loss is greater than the 20 per cent drop seen after the natural or premature menopause (when the ovaries continue to produce androgens).[15] However, the evidence that these hormonal changes are linked to libido is mixed.

Women can keep menopausal symptoms at bay and reduce their longer-term risks by using HRT within days of their surgery. In the UK women who have had a hysterectomy as well as an oophorectomy are prescribed oestrogen-only HRT; those with wombs receive combined HRT. Sometimes gynaecologists suggest an HRT implant during surgery so the patient has time to recover before deciding which HRT to use. This choice appeals to some women; others prefer to start with tablets or patches, which can be changed easily if side-effects cause trouble or, much more rarely, the original health problem is reactivated.

The question of reactivation is likely to concern women with endometriosis, not least because the patient leaflets in HRT packs advise them to mention this history to their doctors. Endometriosis is an oestrogen-dependent condition and therefore there is a possibility that HRT can cause a recurrence of the disease, although the risk is small (5 per cent of cases).[16] The need for blanket caution in drug company literature has been questioned by some researchers who comment that the risk of recurrence may depend on the type of HRT used.[17] They suggest using low doses of natural oestrogens *with* progestogen or perhaps testosterone, rather than synthetic oestrogen or unopposed conjugated equine oestrogens, which have been linked to reported cases of recurrence.

Gynaecologists can also advise women with severe endometriosis to go through a surgical menopause and remain oestrogen-free for a while in the hope of 'starving' the endometriosis (see Angela, below), although the merits of this have not been studied. Others recommend trying tibolone (Livial) in the event of recurrence. One might suppose that the new 'designer' oestrogens (SERMs, see page 72) could offer a solution here because they do not affect the lining of the womb. However, it is not clear how useful they will be in this case because they offer bone protection, but do not reduce menopausal symptoms.

There is little detailed research on whether HRT can alter the risk of recurrence of ovarian cancer, partly because answering such a question requires long-term follow-up of a lot of patients and the disease is uncommon. One of the few studies, which is often quoted, looked back at patients' records and reported that women with ovarian cancer on HRT were more likely to survive a year after hospital presentation than those with the disease who were not on HRT. However, this finding was *not* statistically significant and therefore it may have occurred by chance or been due to other differences between women in the groups, apart from whether they used HRT. Also, the study only looked at what happened during the first year. The authors concluded that HRT didn't present a danger to women with ovarian cancer and could offer quality of life and longer-term protection against problems such as osteoporosis and heart disease.[18] This remains the general medical view to date.

Women who have an oophorectomy may be offered testosterone replacement therapy to remedy any lack of sex drive. It is true that testosterone levels fall more during a surgical menopause, but the few notable studies on testosterone therapy have had mixed results. For example, one controlled study found that oestrogen/testosterone replacement improved libido as measured by reported sexual desire and the frequency of fantasies, improvements which were not seen in women who received oestrogen-only or a placebo after oophorectomy.[19] Nevertheless, this did not lead to significant differences in the number of times women had sex or orgasms, underlining the importance of other influences and the difficulty of defining libido.

This study has also been questioned because women were given doses of testosterone that led to blood levels well above those usually found in pre-menopausal women and such high doses are associated with masculinizing side-effects.[20] There is some evidence that side-effects are dose-related, but it is not clear whether reducing the dose also reduces the reported benefits. Further research is needed, but, in the meantime, women may be offered testosterone replacement on an experimental basis. If they wish to try it, they should check what is being recommended and how their doctor plans to monitor their treatment (see Jane, Chapter 1 and Juanita, Chapter 6). The types of testosterone HRT available and likely follow-up tests vary from country to country.

Ironically, until fairly recently most women having an early oophorectomy were faced with an untreated surgical menopause. For example, a 1989 study found only 23 per cent of patients under the age of 40 were offered HRT and frequently treatment only lasted for an average of 28 months.[21] This is not long enough to gain later protection from heart disease and osteoporosis. The UK National Osteoporosis Society (NOS) reports that 25 per cent of its members with severe osteoporosis had a hysterectomy and/or oophorectomy before their natural menopause, and three-quarters of these women were never advised to take HRT.[22] Views have changed: in a recent British survey 99 per cent of consultants agreed that HRT was advisable after surgical menopause, as long as a woman's medical history wasn't against it, and 27 per cent would contemplate *indefinite* treatment.[23]

Nowadays women are often prescribed HRT during their hospital stay, a time when they are receiving specialist medical attention. However, unless they are due to have further monitoring (e.g. after ovarian cancer), women are unlikely to see the prescribing doctor again. This means that even those who felt well-advised about their illness and treatment can be surprised by the uncertainty of their follow-up care on HRT (see Jane, Chapter 1). Women may assume that regular prescriptions mean some kind of check-up (as they do on the Pill), only to find that this depends on their local general practice and/or their GP's knowledge and interest in HRT.

The British survey of GPs and gynaecologists was not reassuring about follow-up care: 'significant numbers of both groups failed to answer questions relating to investigating and monitoring [HRT]'. Since then the Royal College of Obstetricians and Gynaecologists (RCOG), Royal College of General Practitioners (RCGP) and National Osteoporosis Society have produced a formal statement, which urges hospital and general practice staff to 'provide advice on HRT . . . to all women who have had a hysterectomy before the natural menopause' and notes that such women 'require regular monitoring'.[24] It is less clear what this monitoring should involve or how regularly women should be seen.

Oophorectomy is usually accompanied by hysterectomy, but younger women may be given the chance to retain some of their eggs and/or their wombs. If eggs can be removed and fertilized by their partner's sperm before surgery, the resultant embryos will be frozen until the patient is ready to attempt pregnancy. Usually, single women are not able to keep theirs eggs because suitable techniques for freezing and thawing unfertilized eggs are still being developed. Alternatively a woman may be able to keep her womb in the hope of later egg-donation IVF (see Teresa, below). Other women will not have this opportunity or will feel unable to take up fertility treatment for religious or ethical reasons. Young women who have full surgery may plan to adopt instead (see Lynnette, below), or find other ways to have children in their lives or express their creativity.

Medical Menopause

The medical menopause is caused by cancer treatments such as radio- or chemotherapy, which damage the egg follicles in the ovaries. This can be a problem for young women diagnosed with cancers such as Hodgkin's disease or non-Hodgkin's lymphoma, leukaemia and related disorders, and some childhood cancers.

Cancer treatments are designed to disrupt cells that are multiplying rapidly. They can also affect a cell's DNA (genetic instructions). This makes them good at targeting cancer cells, although other sensitive cells will be affected as well. Usually the body can renew these, but the ovaries' store of egg follicles is formed before birth and cannot be replaced. As described in Chapter 2, each follicle is a large collection of cells that surrounds an egg. When follicles are activated during the menstrual cycle, these cells multiply to several million to feed the egg and orchestrate its release. This rapid division makes active follicles vulnerable to chemotherapy, but treatment may also disrupt the DNA in inactive follicles.[25] If too many follicles are damaged, the woman concerned will lose her fertility and ability to make oestrogen and progesterone. Her menstrual cycle will come to an end, followed by menopausal symptoms and an increased risk of osteoporosis and heart disease in later years.

However, sometimes the body can reverse an apparent medical menopause. Indeed, the younger a woman is during chemotherapy, the greater the chances of her ovaries withstanding treatment or recovering. For example, younger women continue to have periods on a higher average total dose of cyclophosphamide compared to older women. There appears to be a similar age effect for radiotherapy: younger women's periods are more likely to resume naturally, in time.

There are even reports of women becoming pregnant years later (with no extra risk to the baby). This difference seems to be related to the greater number of follicles in younger women's ovaries. It is as if they can bear losing follicles during treatment because they have more to begin with. This can be very good news for patients in their teens and twenties, but is less reassuring for somewhat older women.

Researchers have looked at whether treatment can be improved so that the ovaries are protected. For example, ovarian failure is usually inevitable with radiotherapy doses above 800 rads, but can be avoided using 150 rads or less.[26] Such damage is also less likely if treatment is further away from the ovaries. Of course, the area exposed and dose used are often dictated by the type and stage of disease being treated, so the radiotherapy may not remain effective if it is changed. Doctors have tried other ways of protecting the ovaries, such as moving them out of the way surgically (without disrupting their blood supply). This requires a major operation (laparotomy), although it may become possible using key-hole surgery (laparoscopy). Researchers have also investigated whether drugs that shut down the ovaries temporarily can make them less vulnerable to radiation, although they have not had much success.[27]

Women and girls with leukaemia and related disorders can be treated with bone-marrow transplant after total body irradiation and/ or chemotherapy. In this case, the ovaries are unlikely to recover, whether the bone-marrow transplant involves cyclophosphamide alone or in conjunction with total body irradiation.[28] Nowadays, as with pre-menopausal women about to undergo an oophorectomy or hysterectomy, women with partners may be invited to save some of their eggs before such treatment begins in order that embryos may be frozen and stored until they are ready to manage a pregnancy (see Andrea, below).

Women faced with a medical menopause are usually treated with combined HRT, rather than oestrogen-only HRT, because they have their wombs. This will reduce their menopausal symptoms and the extra risks of osteoporosis and heart disease. HRT will not reactivate cancers such as Hodgkin's disease, non-Hodgkin's lymphoma and leukaemia because they are not oestrogen-dependent diseases. However, once cancer treatment is complete, women may find that they share questions about HRT and their follow-up care with younger women who lack ovarian hormones for other reasons.

Women's Stories

Betty (Australia)

I had normal periods before having my first child at 26 and my second at 29. A few years later, I found my periods were getting longer and much closer together. Eventually I went to the doctor who put me on the Pill. I don't know the medical name, but in those days not many were available.

I was very depressed, quick-tempered and unhappy on the Pill. In retrospect, I think it was a mental attitude to the Pill, feeling I shouldn't be taking something to stop children. We had other precautions re birth control and, while we didn't really want another child, we felt it was more in God's hands than ours.

I returned to the doctor and told him my side-effects. He said, 'You're "real bitchy"' (I'll never forget his words as that described what I was like). An op was arranged. I had fibroids and damaged ovaries, so had a full hysterectomy at 39. Physically I recovered quickly, but mentally it took some years. I cried because I couldn't have any more children (even though I had two and didn't really want more). I couldn't look at, nurse or talk to babies for quite some time. There was no help from any support group. My husband was great and in time I got over it.

I was also on HRT tablets, which I took once a day for 10 years, until I turned 50. Then my doctor said there was a risk of breast cancer and decided to take me off them. I started having hot flushes, but not too badly, so stayed off anything till I was 64. By then I'd read so much on older women on HRT that I asked my doctor if I should be on it. I'd also broken my leg a few years before, so she suggested a bone-density test. The results showed I had osteoporosis, so she prescribed Premarin (0.625 mg) to try and stop it getting worse. I have to go for another bone-density test this year to see if the Premarin has slowed it down. I was told it could, but wouldn't cure the damage already done. I have no side-effects or problems now and feel very well.

In my day not enough was known of these drugs and also I had to have my husband sign a consent form for the hysterectomy because, at 39, I was considered to be still of child-bearing age. Things are different today – women make their own decisions, which is as it should be.

Teresa

My troubles began two years ago, aged 27. I visited my GP complaining of deep abdominal pains (not unlike 'stitch'). He said he couldn't find anything physically wrong and put my pains down to Fallopian tube spasm and I was to live with it unless it got worse.

Six months later, I fell from a horse. The next two months were hell. At the start of my periods I suffered even worse pains, nausea and dizziness. I saw a woman GP, who agreed something was wrong and referred me to a gynaecologist.

My gynaecologist said he felt something wrong with my ovaries, possibly growths. I had repeated ultrasound scans which showed the cysts were growing. Eventually it was decided that an operation was necessary. I lost my left ovary to a 10 cm cyst and half my right ovary to a biocular [double] cyst, 7.5 cm and 5 cm. After the initial recovery (I was black and blue), I felt better than I had done for years. But I had a post-operative check-up after six weeks and was told my remaining ovary felt enlarged. More ultrasound scans followed and, yes, there was yet another cyst and it was growing.

I was asked if I wanted to try and grow some eggs, but I refused. The chances of actually harvesting viable eggs were slight as my ovaries were producing cysts, and I felt I'd had too many disappointments already. Also, we felt that having fertilized eggs stored for future use would put us under the added pressure of a finite time limit to have a family – and if we didn't and the eggs had to be destroyed, then we would be responsible for killing the life (lives) we had started. I believe it is life the moment eggs are fertilized, and that would have been too much for me to bear.

Four months later I returned to hospital to have my right ovary removed. I'd tried to keep it. My gynaecologist did his utmost to save it, but it just wasn't to be.

I'd had time to think and talk to my husband, time to prepare, or so I thought. But nothing could have prepared me for the trauma. I had a whole range of feelings and thoughts. Those of anger, grief and emptiness and that old chestnut, 'why me?' To say I hit rock-bottom was an understatement. My husband, family and friends rallied round and offered me their love and support. They told me I was still me and at least it wasn't life threatening and, yes, I know it could have been much worse. I knew that, but it didn't help. I felt as though I was half a woman, unable to conceive. I felt immensely guilty; I'd let everyone down: me, my husband, his family (he's an only child). I think the guilt is the worst thing, I'm still learning to live with it. One day I hope the hurt will be less.

Another aspect, of course, is the HRT. I feel women should be better informed about what is involved so we know what to expect. I opted to take tablets. I started on Climagest 1 mg. I didn't feel right, so the dose was increased to 2 mg. I felt better in some ways, but I was getting severe PMT and mood swings that frightened me, never mind my poor husband. I also had awful headaches. I told my GP and she changed me to Femoston 2/10, the PMT did ease, but I felt like my batteries were draining, so now I'm on Femoston 2/20. I expected to be given the right dose immediately and all would be perfect. No, it seems it's all trial and error until you happen on the right one.

As for IVF, I would need a donor egg now. I have the greatest respect for egg donors; they give the gift of hope to women like myself. At present I don't feel emotionally strong enough to attempt IVF. It's only been 10 months since my last operation. Maybe given time, I just don't know yet.

My husband has been an absolute rock, giving his support and taking the brunt of my moods, my anger, my loss, and he constantly reminds me that there's so much to life, that we can share our lives and go on from there. Sometimes I can't help wondering what a child of mine would have looked like, but it is something I'll never know.

Angela

I had 'chocolate' ovarian cysts and severe widespread endometriosis stuck to my bowel, bladder, etc., most of which couldn't be removed. The cervix was completely stuck down, which is why I had a sub-total hysterectomy and bilateral oophorectomy – they just couldn't remove my cervix. Apparently I signed a consent form, but no one mentioned the possibility of such drastic surgery to me beforehand or its implications, e.g. instant surgical menopause and at the age of just 31!! Amazing, isn't it, and all without informed consent!

I was advised by my consultant not to take HRT for a year post op, as it could cause the endometriosis, which couldn't be removed, to grow back. During that time things were pretty bad and I was on anti-depressants and sleeping tablets. Without HRT the menopausal symptoms were horrendous and began almost immediately after my surgery with hot flushes, insomnia, early-morning waking, fatigue and depression. The effects of surgical menopause hadn't been discussed with me in detail while in hospital, so I wasn't prepared for the severity of these symptoms. It was a very difficult time and I couldn't wait to start HRT, which, I was given the impression, would solve all my problems and everything would be wonderful from then on.

A year later I began oestrogen replacement therapy, first Progynova tablets, then Harmogen tablets (which both made me nauseous), then Evorel patches, but it was soon apparent that the endometriosis had grown back as the pain and some bleeding began all over again. My doctor told me this was because the oestrogen had reactivated the endometriosis deposits that were impossible to remove during surgery, especially in the cervix, which couldn't be removed as it would have been in a normal hysterectomy. I had an ultrasound to check it wasn't anything more sinister and was then prescribed Provera tablets to suppress the endometriosis. This caused a lot of sudden weight gain, so after five months I stopped taking that also. Luckily by then the bleeding had stopped, but I still had the pain.

Being worried about osteoporosis as I'm so young (now 34), I had a bone-density scan, which showed osteopenia (mild osteoporosis). My doctor refused to pay for the scan and so I paid for it myself. Not wanting oestrogen because of the fear of endometriosis, I am taking Didronel only now. However, not being on HRT, I still have unacceptable menopausal symptoms such as insomnia and feeling very, very hot day and night. So much so that I haven't felt able to work for the last two years and, after leaving my job, went back into full-time, and then part-time education. I tried soya milk, phytoestrogen bread and a herbal remedy called Remifemin (made from black cohosh, which I got from Germany), but nothing seems to help and I feel just as bad.

My doctor wants me to go back on HRT, but I just can't decide. My consultant doesn't seem interested. Luckily I have Internet access at home and I have been gathering information as much as possible about my options. I've also joined several Internet mailing lists such as Sans-uteri, Menopaus List, Witsendo [see More Help] and more recently a UK-based list for menopause sufferers called Curses [now discontinued]. They have all been very informative, especially Sans-uteri, without which I think I would have gone mad by now!! I've made several 'e-pals' all over the world and we keep in touch on a regular basis, giving each other much-needed emotional support as we are all in similar situations.

I would like some specialist help and am trying to find out if I can be referred to a menopause clinic or a gynaecological endocrinologist. Being in my thirties, I am worried about what the future holds, whether I choose to take HRT again or not.

Clair

For the past 15 years, I have just accepted HRT as a necessary part of my life. The alternative at the time of my hysterectomy was unacceptable – sudden and complete menopause aged 30. Now I am beginning to question whether enough is being done to research the long-term effects of HRT.

At 24, after years of pain and illness, I had an ovary removed during an emergency operation for a burst ovarian cyst, but continued to suffer for three years until another emergency laparotomy established the problem was endometriosis. After six more operations, I had a hysterectomy and the other ovary removed.

Although my gynaecologist was excellent, no time was allocated by him or other staff for counselling – I was 30, divorced, childless and HRT was really only just beginning to come into general use. I knew no one else receiving hormone treatment and feared I would become some sort of horrible monster through its side-effects! The gynaecologist assured me it was safe, but the few weeks before receiving HRT were so dreadful with the immediate onset of meno-pausal symptoms that I was willing to take anything.

It was about a year before I found HRT that suited me. I tried several, including a pack with one tablet for 21 days/another for seven days (this caused the most appalling mood swings), an implant twice (I didn't like being subjected to little cuts, I was scarred enough already!) and eventually settled to Premarin 1.25 mg per day. Almost immediately I realized this was best. I have no mood swings. I feel healthy, energetic and pain free and have taken it for all the years since. The only side-effect was weight gain and increase in breast size, which was a small penalty for the overall gains.

Since then I have moved around a lot and each GP has continued prescribing Premarin without question. Until recently, when my local surgery sorted out their computer system, no one had been pro-active in suggesting regular checks – blood pressure, etc. – but everyone has been happy to do so when asked. After hearing in the press about the small increase in breast-cancer risk, I consulted my GP about this and the effects of long-term HRT. He reassured me that this was outweighed by the positive reduction in the risk of heart disease.

On the sexual side, the hysterectomy did cause a significant drying of my vagina (but this can always be treated by creams) and a slight reduction in libido. However, I enjoy a full and satisfying sex life and again these are small problems that I have gladly accepted in order to be well.

I have to say that I am probably one of the 'success' stories. I am healthy, happy, extremely active, have no mood swings, my blood pressure is excellent and whether due to HRT or family genes, I look young for my age! I am now married and, through my husband, surrounded by children.

I do hope doctors will give room for counselling women who suffer early menopause for whatever reason, especially those who are childless. The need for understanding is ongoing, for we are always 'out of step' with our peer group – childless when friends are pregnant, no PMT when friends are suffering, no menopause when colleagues are bemoaning their symptoms and no grandchildren when our friends are delighting in theirs!

Lynnette

My husband and I had been trying for a family for two years, so I decided to see my GP. I was 24. I saw a gynaecologist who diagnosed an ovarian cyst the size of a pineapple. He said I would need this removed, but it wasn't anything to worry about. I hadn't had any symptoms other than feeling bloated now and again and going to the toilet more often – I just put this down to 'women's things'.

He sent me for an ultrasound scan, then a CAT scan. This showed I had a cyst on the other ovary too, wrapped round my bowel. By this time I was starting to get worried, but tried to put any scary thoughts to the back of my mind.

A week went by before I was admitted to hospital. At last, I thought, this operation will enable me to have the children we both long for – how wrong I was.

I had the op in early December four years ago. The next day I was feeling sore and groggy, but not too bad. The gynaecologist came to see me, drew the curtains round the bed and sat down to say that he'd had to give me a full hysterectomy due to ovarian cancer in both ovaries. He said he was so sorry, but he'd had only a few minutes to make this decision. I remember the first thing I said was, 'I'd rather die than go through what my sister went through.'

I was utterly devastated, all hopes of being a mother had gone within 24 hours and I had to face cancer as well. When I first saw my husband and Mam, I just didn't know where to start. Telling them was one of the hardest things I've had to do, especially after we'd been down this road before with my sister (although not with ovarian cancer). We all cried together.

As I lay in bed, all I could hear going through my head was 'I've got cancer, I've got cancer'. I waited for two days for the lab results – what long days they were. The results were between borderline and Stage 1. I sobbed with relief, they had caught it early.

Five days after the op I was given Carboplatin. This made me feel sick but it was OK. It was during these few days that I first experienced hot flushes and night sweats. My hormones had gone from normal to nil during my operation. I wasn't allowed to start HRT until after my first check-up.

I went to stay with my parents. It gave me time to think. I still felt a woman but found it hard to come to terms with not being able to have children and it was the most miserable Christmas I have ever had. I couldn't have got through it without my husband and parents, especially Mam because she had been through this with my sister six months earlier and we had lost that battle.

During this time I was up and down. Panicking because I thought I should get my affairs in order and make a will, but determined I wasn't going to die – I was never offered any counselling or put in touch with any organizations. I had a lot of hot flushes. The night sweats were also uncomfortable. I would wake up with the sheets and my nightie wet with sweat. This was a lot to take in. I was only 24 (my Mam hadn't gone through the menopause, so I couldn't ask her for any advice!) and I felt vulnerable.

I had my first check-up mid-January. My consultant said everything looked to be OK, I was healing nicely and should be able to go back to work at the end of the month. He prescribed Premarin tablets

(0.625 mg daily), said to take this straight away and I would probably be on HRT until I was at least 60! I came away forgetting to ask some of my most important questions: Will I age overnight? What is the risk of breast cancer that I had read about in the papers if you are on HRT for more than 10 years? Do I risk heart disease and osteoporosis if I don't take HRT? And what is in the space where my womb used to be?

With HRT my symptoms took about two weeks to clear up and I started to feel better. Over the next few months I seemed to live between check-ups. I felt I couldn't plan ahead or have a holiday just in case something turned up at a check-up, but gradually I became more positive.

Being on HRT I think has made my hair and skin drier and I get the odd headache, which I think is caused by HRT; I also get thrush, which I never suffered from before – apart from that I'm fine. I still have six-monthly check-ups and, having waited two years, my husband and I have recently adopted a baby girl. So there is happiness at the end after all, even though you think there never will be.

Frances

Many of my friends are older than me and I'd heard discussions about menopausal symptoms and so on for several years without really listening, thinking it was all some way off. I wanted to have a child at some point, but also felt very ambivalent about it, which is probably why I still didn't have children at 41 when I was diagnosed with Stage 4 ovarian cancer. I'd had a recent, unplanned, ectopic pregnancy and was wondering about a 'last minute' attempt when I became ill.

I asked whether or not eggs could be saved, but was told this procedure takes some months and it wasn't safe to wait before operating. They didn't know whether my ovaries would produce any viable eggs anyway. I was never prepared to risk my life in order to be a mother.

Only one ovary was removed at my first operation, partly because the second looked normal and partly because doctors wanted to see if I would respond to chemotherapy before making me menopausal (quality-of-life issues, they called it). After successful chemotherapy, I asked them to remove the second ovary. The surgeon said it still looked normal on a scan and they were always sorry to remove a healthy ovary from a fertile woman. But I wanted it out. They were all very surprised when lab tests showed it was cancerous. I still have my uterus.

I didn't do anything about HRT immediately because I was going to have more treatment and I thought my body had enough to cope with without further interventions. Everyone said the surgical menopause would probably be instant and dramatic, but I didn't have any symptoms at all for several weeks, and then only a few mild hot flushes. I did notice the flushes got worse when I was stressed. The only other symptom was a dry vagina, which wasn't pleasant, but cancer, surgery, chemo and grief meant that we weren't much interested in sex.

I didn't have particular mood swings, but who can tell what was causing what and what was going on in my mind and body? During the months of surgery and chemotherapy, I lost my father to bowel cancer, about two years after my mother's death from kidney cancer. And there I was, heartbroken, watching my father die, unable to share in caring for him because I was too ill, wondering if the same was going to happen to me. I was also waiting for further experimental treatment (high-dose chemotherapy with stem-cell transplant) and having all sorts of preparatory tests (heart function, kidney function, teeth, hearing and HIV tests, stem-cell growth injections, daily blood tests, stem-cell 'harvesting' and 'priming'). I was medical and research material, but they were saving my life, so I was supposed to be grateful rather than terrified and horrified. The menopause didn't seem like such a big deal.

After the last treatment, I thought about HRT and wasn't sure what to do. I have moved in mainly radical feminist circles, but haven't on the whole shared the widespread belief that conventional medicine is the enemy. I did, however, start to read feminist books on HRT and their analysis made sense to me: that, like childbirth, the menopause has been turned into a medical problem when it is completely natural, may not be a problem at all and, if it is, can be dealt with naturally. My surgeon was very keen to start me on HRT and assumed I would agree. I was worried about the risk of breast cancer, but he said that, at my age, breast tissue expects to be surrounded by oestrogen and it doesn't become a risk until after 'normal' menopausal age.

I opted for HRT, having weighed up the risks, as far as I can. Nobody seems to know much either about ovarian cancer or HRT and I can't, in fact, make a truly 'informed' choice about what to do. As with so many aspects of the disease and treatment, I feel like a guinea pig, trying something but not really knowing what it is doing to me, which makes me uneasy. I have put my trust in my doctors and if they suspect that HRT might help and is unlikely to damage me, this will do for now. Other women I know have made a different choice.

I started using combined patches (Estracombi) and gradually the flushes stopped and lubrication returned. The patches are a constant visible reminder of my situation, which I don't like, but then I don't like my scars either. I have definitely put on weight – but I'm not vain enough to chop and change medications at this point. What may make me change my mind is any change in my health. I see my decisions about HRT as temporary and connected to ongoing reflection and information. I don't know how long I'll stay with it.

The consultant said that maybe five years down the line, I could be a candidate for egg donation. I liked this suggestion because he assumed I had a future, but it didn't occur to me to take it seriously. I don't want to be an elderly mother; I don't trust my health and I don't want to bring a child into our lives with illness hovering. I don't know how I'll feel as time goes on and I don't want to prejudge this, but I simply can't see beyond my struggle for survival yet.

Nearly two years have passed and I am back at work, teaching and writing, but nothing is quite the same. I have constant hospital check-ups and my recovery has not been/is not being smooth: I have worrying blood tests, worrying scans, extra investigations. While there is no visible evidence of disease, there are indications that all is not well. I can never just forget my cancer and move on. I go through periods of intense sorrow and I have become more, not less, broody and sad that I can never be a mother. I am so sad and bewildered by what has been happening to me and just wonder why I have not been allowed to have a 'normal' life, which everyone else seems to take for granted.

I am grateful, however, that these moments do pass and that I am generally quite strong-willed and very determined to survive. Menopause really is the least of my worries – I want to enjoy my life, be with the people I love, do the things I love doing and not become overwhelmed by the unfairness of it or by the fear of what I may yet have to face. I spend much of my time not thinking about it; my main concern is to manage the anxiety, find a balance between my various activities (work, rest and play), rethink my career and relationships and try to get things as right as possible.

Ali

I am 38, but have been 'menopausal' for half my life. But have I? So many of our expectations of the menopause are bound up with the nature of age and ageing and conventional views of what women will do in their lives. None of those things fit my circumstances.

In 1977, aged 18, I was diagnosed as having Hodgkin's disease. It was like entering a foreign country with no language skills and no interpreter. I did what I was told by those who knew the language and made the rules.

I had a splenectomy and laparotomy. I started mild chemotherapy, but it wasn't working, so I started a course of radiotherapy. I did not have the emotional vocabulary to deal properly with any of this and just got on with it at a shallow level. The radiotherapy was in two batches. I had my 'top half' done first and then had a month off to recover before treatment over my 'lower half'.

During this time, my friend Kathy asked about my womb and ovaries because surely they would be irradiated along with everything else? I rang the hospital. The professor said hadn't the radiologist spoken to me about this? No. Yes, my ovaries could be affected and why not come in and discuss what to do. I did not feel anything at this point because I did not know the implications or what I was supposed to feel. I went in and the radiologist said, 'You are 18, unmarried and we didn't think you'd be too concerned about losing your ovaries.'

Later I also found out that an 'unfortunate mistake' had been made during my laparotomy. Normally they move the ovaries to shield them a bit if radiotherapy is likely. They hadn't, either because they forgot or, at the time, they thought I had an early stage of Hodgkin's and wouldn't need radiotherapy. I would not have refused treatment for the sake of my ovaries – my life is more important – but I feel there was a lack of thought, a lack of care.

My treatment continued and was eventually successful, but only after a year of very gruesome chemotherapy (which in itself would have made me infertile). At some point I had tests, which showed that I had no/not enough oestrogen (to no one's surprise). Although I had hospital check-ups, I don't remember them organizing any HRT. Later I had appointments with a gynaecologist (at an antenatal clinic, of all places) who gave me oestrogen implants for several years (this was before they knew about not giving oestrogen alone if you have a womb). I remember appreciating the difference HRT made to hot flushes, but I still didn't know what was 'normal'.

In 1986 I moved and was prescribed Prempak for many years. Prempak was a misery. I have vivid memories of hating those brown progesterone pills (little brown pills leave me undone) and the hot flushes, depression and almost manic mood swings that I (and friends and colleagues!) had to put up with. When I tried to discuss this, the doctor was unhelpful to the point of rudeness. Once he left the room rather than answer a question. On an earlier occasion, this doctor examined me internally and said, talking to himself, 'Hmm, quite extensive atrophy here.' What young woman wants that kind of comment passed on her?

Eventually I was transferred to a clinic where more people seem to know what they are doing. But no one is concerned with my experiences of HRT – as long as it is fulfilling its basic function.

I now take Premarin and a progesterone called Duphaston (dydro-gesterone). This has been an improvement for several years, but is still not ideal. Today (the sixth of 10 progesterone days), I feel immensely stiff and creaky, as if all my joints have lost their lubrica-tion. I have noticed this often on progesterone. I will have one day of intense lower back pain, for the sake of a minuscule amount of rusty blood (contained by two mini-tampons). I will not call these 'periods' because I do not want to pretend that my menstrual cycle is anything like 'normal'.

Progesterone is the problem. I would be more cheerful on a purely oestrogen day. It's like living with an alcoholic: the problem is worse when the alcoholic is drunk. When they are sober they are still an alcoholic, but it's a relief to be able to forget it and enjoy the sobriety. Until the next time. On oestrogen days I can forget about progesterone, but even on oestrogen days I am infertile and a doctor might say 'atrophy' when he looks at my fanny.

I have tried to experiment with different regimes I've read about, but, without enough support from my GP or any from my consultant, it proved too difficult. The six weeks without oestrogen while I tried to get a prescription for something else sent me sweating back to Premarin.

For several years I was clinically depressed. As well as being in therapy, I took antidepressants (and would recommend them to anyone in that position). I noticed a relationship between progesterone and depression: they worsened each other. Is this just me?

I have had plenty of time to think about the issue of fertility. My fertility – my lack of fertility – is much wider than not being able to have children. As a US artist said, 'Whether we are weaving tissue in the womb or pictures in the imagination, we create out of our bodies'.[29] I think, perhaps, that not being able to 'create' a child has increased my yearning to create other things, to be fertile in other areas. I know that being infertile has shaped me. It has complicated the expression of my sexuality, it has dulled my self-image, and it still hampers and stultifies my creativity.

This is, I have learned, hard for people to understand. Infertile friends seem like kindred spirits until assisted fertilization or adoption, thankfully, brings them children. Then their need is apparently met and they see themselves differently, even though their biological fertility is no different from how it was.

If I were ever to have a child (through egg donation or adoption), I don't know how my fertility feelings would be affected, but I know they would not go away.

I have a big belly and try to reduce it at the gym and by eating well. But should I forgive myself for my slack stomach muscles? Perhaps I would if I was a more typical menopausal age. Things like this are the hardest. I don't know anyone my age who has been on HRT for such a long time. Am I as I am because I am menopausal or because I am a not-very-fit 38-year-old? What is normal for 38? What is normal for someone who is 38 but has been on HRT for 20 years?

Andrea

I began to feel quite unwell about four years ago. I picked up a cough and a cold, which I just couldn't seem to get rid of, and began to feel very tired, especially as coughing kept me awake most nights. I was also having the most unusual periods. Some of them lasted all month and then, other months, I wouldn't have a period at all! I must admit that I attributed my condition to the problems in my life at the time. I had recently separated from my husband (the most unpleasant experience) and I was closing the shop I managed, making redundant and retiring my staff. My own career was also looking a bit unstable. In addition, I was in the penultimate year of a distance-learning degree. So, as you can see, life was pretty busy. However, on the plus side I had recently met a lovely man, Alan, who unbeknown to me, was to provide me with one very important reason for living.

That March, I visited my doctor for an insurance-policy medical. My family has a history of Huntingdon chorea and, although it hasn't manifested itself in the last two generations, I knew this was the reason for the medical. I arrived at my doctor's feeling OK and left feeling like I had one foot in the grave! He said that I had a heart murmur, was anaemic, had low blood pressure and that he wanted me to have a hospital blood test. Well, one blood test followed another and in June my doctor recommended a bone-marrow test. I asked if there was anything to worry about, and he said no, not really, because he didn't think it was leukaemia.

To cut a long story short, I did in fact have a rare form of leukaemia called myelodysplasia, which is particularly difficult to treat. As the disease was evolving, my consultant suggested a bone-marrow transplant. There was enough understanding of the disease to know that chemotherapy would not provide a cure. This meant that I needed a donor. After much tissue matching, my brother was found to be a good source. This was a major triumph because it meant I had some chance of survival. Over the next month we agreed a drug protocol with the consultants. I would have total body irradiation followed by two or three lots of chemotherapy and then a bone-marrow transplant. I would also be given norethisterone (which gave me awful stomach cramps) to stop me menstruating when I had the transplant.

On Wednesday July 27th Alan took me shopping and asked me to choose a ring. That evening he asked me if I would like to go to the beach. We live quite near the sea and had spent several evenings there just enjoying each other's company. This time Alan packed his guitar and a bottle of red wine and we headed off just before midnight. Although I had seen a ring I liked, I did not realize that Alan had gone and bought it. So I could not believe it when he got down on one knee and asked me to marry him. Of course, I said yes and we came to an agreement that we would get married when I got better!

As the days went by it began to dawn on me that I might not be able to have children as a result of my treatment. Nobody had explicitly mentioned it, but common sense was beginning to kick in. Eventually, and after many highs and lows, we were given the chance to try the latest technology and yet again I was to become something of a scientific breakthrough. I was the first person, certainly in South-ampton and possibly in England, to have the opportunity to freeze embryos ready for implantation after cancer. Until then doctors had been able to freeze sperm, but there was no option available for women. We heard the wonderful news about IVF on September 2nd, but as I was due to start the total body irradiation on October 10th, I had just one go at IVF. We were very lucky and now have seven embryos, stored and waiting.

Unfortunately my bone-marrow transplant did not work. As soon as my blood count started to come back we knew almost straight away that the treatment had not been successful. I still had some of my own bone-marrow cells left and we knew that it would only be a matter of time before I developed acute myeloid leukaemia. My consultant and I continued trying different treatments during the following year, but by the next September I had developed leukaemia. At this stage there was only a 5 per cent chance of a second transplant working and it was unlikely my organs would be strong enough to put up with any more of the graft-versus-host side-effects.

We were running out of treatments when my consultant came back from a conference about a pioneering new treatment and asked me if I would 'like a go'. It involved taking the lymphocytes from my brother's blood and giving them to me. Naturally I accepted and we went ahead on September 25th. Unfortunately this did not work either. At Christmas I went down with pleurisy and by early January the leukaemia had returned. There were three options: do nothing and let the leukaemia take its course, have further chemotherapy (with no realistic chances of cure), or have more chemotherapy with a further donor-lymphocyte infusion. We decided on the third. This meant at least another two large doses of chemo over the next few months (mainly in hospital) and then a donor-lymphocyte infusion. It was touch and go, especially as I caught pneumonia the day I came out of hospital and ended up back in isolation. However, I was out again by the beginning of April and actually managed to attend my graduation ceremony that month.

I have been on HRT (Prempak-C 1.25 mg) since my original transplant three years ago because I am sterile, have suffered the side-effects of the menopause and am likely to get osteoporosis if I don't take HRT. Until I started HRT, I had night sweats that would leave me absolutely soaking and needing to change my night clothes more than once a night. I also had some hot flushes. I don't seem to have many problems on HRT, except that I sometimes have two periods in one month.

I would like a consultation with an experienced gynaecologist to make sure that I am on the correct dose and to discuss the realistic chances of Alan and I starting our family in a year or so's time once we are married. At the moment, though, I am just happy to be alive and am enjoying every day as much as I can. Being ill has also provided me with the opportunity to pursue a career in teaching, a leap I probably would not have made had it not been for my illness.

9

WHY DOCTORS CAN'T AGREE ABOUT HRT
(AND WOMEN CAN'T EITHER)

'We are expected to trust them, accept what they say and act on it. Where does this leave us when doctors say different things about HRT?'

JENNIFER

Researching this book involved attending professional and public meetings to hear medical and other speakers discuss the menopause and HRT. Soon one had heard almost every point of view greeted by both applause and derisory laughter. Clearly doctors did not agree about HRT and women didn't either, although this was more than a doctor:patient divide.

Many of these arguments were about facts and evidence. But frequently they had more to do with the way people saw the menopause. For example, the observation that oestrogen levels largely decline after the menopause was not at stake compared to the meaning of this decline, and hence the implications for 'treatment'. Even doctors were not agreed about whether this meant all women should receive HRT.

This chapter is a brief guide to some of the places people can be coming from in the HRT debate and the grounds for their arguments. It also describes why 'randomized controlled trials' and the 'placebo effect' are recurring themes in disputes about scientific evidence.

The Medical Model of the Menopause

A 'model' is a mental map of reality. A way of making sense of the world. The medical model provides a framework that enables doctors to diagnose disease and treat patients, often to great benefit. It does so by seeing the body in a certain way and from a particular point of view. This outlook extends to the menopause. However, some doctors adopt the medical model of the menopause more completely than others, and one doesn't have to be a doctor to agree with it – or a woman to disagree with it!

In the medical model, natural menopause is seen as a pathological state of oestrogen deficiency. Lack of oestrogen may cause symptoms ranging from hot flushes and vaginal dryness to loss of libido and depression. It is also linked to an increased risk of osteoporosis, heart disease and perhaps Alzheimer's disease. The solution is to replace the missing hormone to treat symptoms and reduce the risks. The parallel often drawn is that of diabetes, where the hormone insulin is replaced to restore health.

Critics argue that the menopause is a natural event due to the ageing process. Most women pass through it without significant problems and without seeking medical advice or relief. Therefore women with low hormone levels are not ill or life-threatened, as a diabetic would be without insulin. Hot flushes are not symptoms of a medical disorder but *experiences* of bodily change. While these experiences may be explained by a reduction in hormones, women are not deficient as such. Nor is this natural reduction necessarily the principal cause of later pathology for most women. In this light, waning hormones do not need 'replacing' because they are not 'missing'. Treatment with hormones is unnecessary, *even if* they happen to be natural oestrogens. The same would be said of using natural progesterone (which is advised according to a separate medical model of progesterone deficiency, although not one accepted by most doctors, see Chapter 11).

Those who support the concept of oestrogen deficiency may agree that the hormonal fall after the menopause is natural. They argue nevertheless that this has become an unnatural state of affairs because women are living longer than Nature intended.[1] Some doctors go as far as disqualifying the menopause as a natural event because all other animals breed until they die.[2] According to these views, modern medicine has outstripped evolution with the result that women can be without hormones for 30–40 years. Therefore HRT is a legitimate and necessary aid.

This rationale has been disputed from several quarters. For example, public health doctors and medical anthropologists point out that changes in women's life expectancy simply reflect improvements in childhood diseases and the risks of childbirth.[3] Statistics showing poor life expectancy in the past disguise the fact that women always had a reasonable chance of living into old age, as long as they survived infancy and motherhood. In that sense there is nothing new about the menopause or women living 30–40 years beyond it. The difference is that *more* of them are doing so.

Likewise, biologists suggest that the menopause may be a useful evolutionary adaptation.[4] At first, it is hard to see how losing fertility could be an advantage. After all, evolutionary theory says that useful adaptations remain when they enable survival so that genes can be passed on to offspring! Nevertheless, each pregnancy and birth is risky, and human babies take a long time to grow up. A mother who loses later fertility may be more likely to survive to protect her existing children into adulthood, when they will have children. This could give her genes the edge.

Such a woman may also be more successful in an evolutionary sense if her menopause frees her to look after nieces and nephews. Biologists point out that experienced parenting can influence the survival of offspring. Furthermore, baby monkeys appear more likely to live when born into an extended family (which includes male care-givers!). Experienced carers who work in a group may be better at forwarding their collective genes, including those that convey the advantage of having a menopause.

Doctors who assert that the menopause is unnatural because animals breed until they die rarely follow this argument to its logical conclusion. Few doctors seek to restore women's fertility at this stage. Indeed, Italian cases of egg-donation IVF in post-menopausal women provoked a medical and public outcry.[5] Restoring older women's hormones is one thing; restoring their fertility seems to be quite another, medically and culturally.

Some doctors have argued that there is no need to see *all* menopausal women as oestrogen deficient in order to help a minority who want relief.[6] This raises the question of who should be treated with HRT. As several researchers asked, 'Is HRT used to treat abnormal conditions (e.g. premature menopause or oophorectomy), is it medication for symptomatic relief (e.g. hot flushes), or is it prophylaxis (preventive treatment) for at-risk groups or for all women?'[7]

A survey of British gynaecologists and GPs showed widespread agreement that 'high-risk' groups, such as women with a family history of osteoporosis or those with premature/surgical menopause, should be prescribed HRT.[8] Fewer felt this should be the case for all eligible women (64 per cent of gynaecologists, 56 per cent of GPs). This uncertainty was seen in another survey of GPs. Fifty per cent agreed that the 'menopause was best seen as an oestrogen-deficiency condition'. Yet 67 per cent disagreed with the statement that 'all women over 45 should be advised to have HRT'.[9] These findings may reflect the extent to which doctors embrace the medical model and their concern about incomplete evidence for the efficacy and safety of long-term HRT. Some doctors are firmly against HRT.[10]

Other 'medical' models of the menopause can be found elsewhere. For example, alternative practitioners often have a 'medical' perception of the problem. That is, the problem is perceived to originate within the body and symptoms dictate the kind of treatment prescribed, even though they may not be defined, diagnosed, explained or treated in the conventional way. Like conventional medicine, this requires expertise. All these models are in contrast to feminist views of the menopause, as the following section shows.

Feminist Arguments

Broadly feminists reject the idea that 'anatomy is destiny' and hence that women's experiences during the menopause are determined primarily by their bodies. Rather, their model is that many so-called symptoms result from the way society – and medicine – views menopausal women. This determines in turn how women come to view themselves.

They point out that society defines and values women in terms of their sexual and reproductive functions as wives and mothers. Medicine defines them by their wayward bodies and raging hormones, which have long been linked to hysteria or insanity and, more recently, to depression and the psychological symptoms of PMT.[11] Seen in this light, menopausal women are by definition sexually and socially redundant, medically and emotionally out of control. It is therefore no accident that the remedy, HRT, claims to restore sexual usefulness, even attractiveness, and provide control against everything from crumbling bones to a crumbling mind.

In this way, the menopause and ageing have been *medicalized*, i.e. changed into disorders to be prevented and treated within the body by medicine. Feminists (and others) contend that this process is widespread. Perhaps their most familiar example is the way childbirth has been turned into a medical event to be attended to by doctors in a medical setting. Another example is the approach to compulsive eating. This has become a medical condition where doctors intervene with psychiatric treatment, lipid-lowering drugs or stomach stapling. In contrast, it is argued that 'fat is a feminist issue'.[12] Compulsive eating – and bulimia and anorexia – is a sign of women's distress in a society that only values those of them who are unrealistically slim and expects women to fulfil the needs of others before their own.

The extent to which society can define 'reality' is illustrated by the experiences of women with intersex conditions [see Chapter 6], whose existence has been denied by a cultural insistence on two separate sexes. (Even recent acknowledgement of transsexuals does not challenge this outlook.) Societies' power to construct alternative views of the menopause is seen in cross-cultural studies. For example, Japanese women do not share the concept of the menopause and the end of menstruation has little cultural significance.[13] Instead they describe *kônenki*, an ageing process linked to the autonomic nervous system rather than oestrogen deficiency.

Feminists comment on how older women in Western society are seen as unappealing, redundant and preferably invisible, and how the media perpetuates this stereotype by focusing almost exclusively on 'young, slim, able-bodied, heterosexual, attractive women'.[14] There is also evidence that negative beliefs about the menopause are common among doctors and women.[15] In keeping with the medical model of unpredictable hormones, it is assumed that women will suffer emotionally as well.

Only recently have women's actual experiences of the menopause been sought in the community (rather than unrepresentative clinics), and studies done to look at social and cultural factors rather than hormones. The research found that, in reality, the menopause is uneventful for most women. Depression was far more strongly associated with personal and social factors, such as negative expectations of the menopause and lack of work outside the home, than whether women were pre- or post-menopausal.[16] This suggests that women need optimistic support and better employment prospects, not HRT. A positive approach may even address the few menopausal symptoms that have been linked to hormone reduction, since the placebo effect for hot flushes is large.[17]

Feminists see the menopause as a political struggle to redefine views of ageing women and their opportunities in life. Some have embraced celebratory images of ageing such as the 'crone' or wise woman. (This may be one reason why feminism is sometimes seen as allied to alternative medicine. In general, however, they argue for empowerment through self-help, information and mutual support rather than seeking authority figures, whether a doctor or alternative expert.) Others have tried to raise awareness of the medicalization of ageing and the dangers of mass hormone treatment, be it with oestrogen, progesterone or testosterone, which have all been equated with 'deficiency' disorders as a rationale for their use. Indeed, even an eminent medical journal has commented that 'universal treatment of a large section of the female population is clearly a glittering prize for the pharmaceutical manufacturer'.[18]

There are signs that feminists may be joined before long by men campaigning against drug treatment of the 'male menopause'. An American specialist in ageing has lamented that 'even though . . . there is no epidemiological, physiological or clinical evidence for such a syndrome, I think . . . the syndrome will [come to] exist. There is a very strong interest in treating ageing men for profit, just as there is for menopausal women.'[19]

Gathering Evidence

Underlying the models are the facts they try to explain. Even with agreed facts, there is plenty of scope for controversy, as the sections above show. But what if even facts cannot be agreed upon? Often this is because of the way 'evidence' was gathered. Here two recurring themes can be heard: randomized controlled trials (RCT) and the placebo effect. The reasons for this provide some insight into arguments about HRT and disputes about alternative treatments. For example, herbalists claim that centuries of traditional practice mean they have no need for randomized trials, but, in the absence of these, doctors can find it difficult to take their assertions seriously. Yet the evidence for HRT is still incomplete.

The prospective randomized controlled trial is thought to provide the best kind of evidence in medical research. A *prospective* study follows people into the future. This is seen as more reliable than investigating past history (retrospective study), which depends on recall, e.g. bad things are often more memorable. A *controlled* trial compares a group who receive treatment with a 'control' group who do not. This supplies information about what could have happened anyway. Then researchers can distinguish whether, for example, the problem improved with treatment or resolved of its own accord.

However, people can also improve because of what is known as the placebo effect.

The placebo effect occurs when people respond to treatment without realizing they have been given an inactive fake (placebo). Perhaps this is 'mind over matter' or the power of positive thinking. Whatever the reason, researchers may draw the wrong conclusion about a treatment's merits unless they take this effect into account. This can be done by comparing a treatment group with a placebo group in a blind trial where participants do not know what they have been allocated.

The placebo effect is very large in women with hot flushes. Dummy pills can provide widespread relief and in some trials the effect is almost as great as HRT. Perhaps this is because the expectation that help is at hand causes relaxation, which reduces hot flushes. Not surprisingly the benefits of many alternative treatments for menopausal symptoms have been put down to the placebo effect by doctors. On an individual level, women may not care one way or the other, as long as they feel better as a result – although they may want to think twice if the remedy is costly or of unknown safety. Equally, if placebos are almost as good as HRT for hot flushes, they may want to opt for relaxation techniques instead of drug treatment! For example, breathing exercises can help hot flushes and women have been trained to reduce these symptoms using cognitive relaxation therapy.[20]

Practitioners' expectations can affect treatment results just as much as patients'. This potential bias can be avoided if the trial is 'double blind'. Here not even the researchers know who is getting dummy therapy until the investigation is decoded at the end. The need to do this is underlined by many a cautionary tale. The following one was repeated recently by way of warning in a medical journal.[21] In 1906 the distinguished scientist Dr Robert Bennett Bean reported his genuine conclusion that white people were more advanced than black people. His assessment was based on ratios calculated from many careful measurements on brains taken from 200 corpses. Yet when the measurements were repeated on the same brains by someone else, no racial distinction could be found. Dr Bean knew whether the brain in front of him was from a black or white person. His successor did not.

This tale is a reminder of feminist arguments that social perceptions can determine the way a problem is defined and evidence seen. It also highlights the need to clarify whether measurements are valid (does brain size equate with intelligence?) and reliable (can they be repeated?). The idea that a ratio of fore- and hind-brain size measures intelligence may be laughable now, but the same questions have to be asked about measures that seem plausible today. Other chapters describe whether, for example, bone density provides a valid and reliable guide to the risk of later fractures and question which bones should be gauged. A similar difficulty is seen in the quarrel about whether blood or saliva tests measure the effects of natural progesterone treatment.

The research techniques described above are used, where possible, to avoid different kinds of bias. Another method is *randomization*. A randomized trial involves allocating women at random (by computer) into the treatment or control group. This rules out the possibility that an unintended difference between the groups will influence the results. For example, doubts were expressed when a large study reported that HRT reduced the risks of heart disease because the participants had already made personal decisions about HRT. Women who choose HRT may be different from those who do not. This could be the reason for their future health, rather than HRT. Nevertheless, asking women to take part in a lottery raises immediate questions, not least whether it is ethical to do so. For this reason randomization may not be an option or, if it is, may be so only after approval from ethics committees.

Even if all these safeguards are in place, a trial that is not large enough may not reveal a statistically significant result. A result is said to be 'significant' when the likelihood of it occurring by chance is less than 5 per cent (and 'very significant' if the likelihood is less than 1 per cent). Here the key words are *by chance*. The idea of a research result occurring by chance may be unfamiliar and yet life is full of chance, chaos even. Take the simple research project of tossing a coin. Heads or tails? The result will be due to chance. But what if one throws surprisingly few heads? Apart from being suspicious, one could do a statistical test that calculates the odds on this result. If heads turn up less than 5 per cent of the time, this is statistically significant, i.e. it is unlikely to have occurred by chance and therefore there may be another explanation. Perhaps the coin is bent.

But which is a better research project: 10 or 1000 throws? The first 10 throws may make one suspicious, but not the second 10. After 100, one might see a trend, but a slight trend may only be clear after 1000 throws. The larger a clinical trial, the more likely it is to detect a significant result, if one exists. A large drug trial also allows risks and benefits to be assessed with greater precision. Yet many studies are said to be 'underpowered' in this respect (rather like the 10 throws).[22] To redress this, data from several comparable studies may be compiled and re-analysed (meta-analysis). Estimates for the extra risk of breast cancer in HRT users aged 50–70 were arrived at in this way (see Figure 5.7, page 96). However, lack of data means that similar estimates are not available for the smaller number of women who lose their hormones at an early age (but see pages 95–7).

These are just some of the reasons why many studies produce results that are open to question and the evidence for HRT is incomplete, even by medical standards. As one reviewer commented, 'It would be wonderful to have to hand the results of at least one randomized prospective trial that evaluated the outcome of treatment in terms of clinical events such as fracture and heart attacks.'[23] The difficulty is that heart attacks, fragility fractures and breast cancer tend to occur many years after the menopause. So studies to look at the effects of HRT *on these problems* are lengthy. Not surprisingly such studies are expensive and difficult to organize, especially as they also require very large numbers to provide reliable statistics. Indeed, the number of women involved means that such projects demand collaboration by several research centres, even countries.[24] This has led researchers to look at the effect of HRT on *risk factors* and estimate the likely result on later disease.

All these limitations fuel the argument about how *much* evidence one needs before it is ethical to prescribe a drug – or unethical not to. The pressures to do so become even greater if it is thought to affect the chances of a major cause of death. With HRT the stakes are high. Those in favour say that doctors should prescribe now because this could prevent heart disease and osteoporosis and make a big difference to the health of women. Those against say not enough is known about the possible risks, and what if the predicted benefits do not come to fruition? The history of HRT has already been marked by overconfidence.

This is where the debate gets into the 'precautionary principle'. It says, 'Where there are significant risks of damage to public health, we should be prepared to take action to diminish those risks, even when the scientific knowledge is not conclusive, if the balance of likely costs and benefits justifies it.'[25] Some doctors see the menopause in just this light, i.e. as oestrogen deficiency that carries 'significant risks of damage' to women's health in later life. They feel HRT should be prescribed to reduce these risks even though current knowledge is incomplete because they regard the balance as in favour of HRT.

Others have argued that the 'risk' approach to the menopause has been invoked for commercial reasons and because of the politics of ageing. One reviewer comments on research that has tracked the 'construction of the menopause as a condition of risk and the marketing of hormones to subvert that risk'.[26] She notes that women are being 'disciplined indirectly' to be virtuous and seek health in countries where ageing populations are likely to prove a burden to the state. Another academic argues that 'the body . . . has become a commodified and regulated object that must be strictly monitored by its owner to prevent lapses into health-threatening behaviour as identified by risk.[27] Put more simply, these arguments suggest it could be a short step to blaming women who do not comply with HRT. What is known as the 'victim-blaming' attitude is already well-established towards smokers, unhealthy eaters and others who appear to be negligent about lifestyle advice, in spite of the powerful commercial lobbies and social pressures that encourage their behaviour.

Many of the arguments described in this chapter have appeared in medical and professional journals and disputes are likely to be ongoing. Various wings of the debate are also reflected in the existence of pro- and anti-HRT doctors' organizations as well as different doctor-led patient information services and campaign groups. Women-led organizations and self-help groups also reflect a range of views. However, as one medical reviewer commented, 'In an ideal world we should not take sides.' He adds, 'For women to benefit from basic and clinical research concerning the menopause, there must be a greater dialogue.'[28]

USING HRT

HRT comes in all shapes and sizes, yet finding the right treatment can be a matter of trial and error. Sometimes it involves changing to a different type to reduce side-effects; sometimes one kind of HRT suits a woman's routines or her feelings about medication. As stories in this book show, practical and emotional issues can make a big difference to women who are living on HRT, whether for a few years to see them through the natural menopause or rather longer.

This chapter is a practical guide to help women find the best type of HRT for them, in consultation with their doctor. It describes everything from tablets, skin patches, body gel and implants to vaginal rings, pessaries and creams and discusses the everyday pros and cons of different forms. It also looks at the practicalities of more experimental treatments such as 'bleed-free' HRT and testosterone therapy.

Oestrogen-only HRT

In the UK oestrogen-only HRT is prescribed for women who do not have a womb, either because they have had a hysterectomy or because they were born without one. Oestrogen is taken continuously using one of the methods described below. Women with a womb can take oestrogen tablets or use oestrogen patches or gel as part of combined HRT.

Oestrogen Tablets

There are numerous brands of HRT tablets, with new ones coming on to the market all the time. Their ingredients are less varied. For example, one of the following compounds may be listed on the packet's information leaflet: oestradiol valerate, micronized oestradiol or piperazine oestrone sulphate. All these ingredients are tackled by the gut and liver, so only a percentage of the drug ever reaches the bloodstream. By the time it does, much of it will have been converted into *oestrone*. It doesn't really matter which of these compounds one takes: they all turn up in the bloodstream as the same thing.[1] Even Hormonin, a combination of oestradiol, oestriol and oestrone, ends up the same way. This explains why the oestrogen levels of women taking tablets cannot be monitored reliably by oestradiol blood tests (unlike implants or patches). If such a check-up is necessary, doctors may try to look at the indirect effects of HRT on FSH levels instead.

Tablets containing the ingredients mentioned above are often called natural oestrogens because they contain or give rise to chemicals that are the same as the oestrogens found naturally in women. Doctors may also emphasize that they are made from plants, although this means that plant compounds found in soybeans or cacti have been chemically converted in a laboratory.

Another common type of tablet, Premarin, contains 'conjugated equine oestrogens', i.e. horse oestrogens. Doctors describe these as natural because their chemical structure is similar to that of human oestrogens and women's bodies react to them almost as if they were the real thing. Nevertheless, women can feel Premarin is produced in a very unnatural way (see Chapter 4).

Some tablets contain a synthetic form of oestrogen, such as ethinyl oestradiol or mestranol. Synthetic oestrogens are more potent than natural oestrogens and can be unnecessarily strong for HRT. For example, ethinyl oestradiol is used in the contraceptive pill to prevent ovulation and pregnancy, whereas oestrogens in HRT are not contraceptive. Since it acts on the relevant hormone receptors, the Pill can be used as a combined form of hormone replacement in younger

Figure 10.1 Examples of the minimum oestrogen doses prescribed to prevent osteoporosis

Tablets   0.625 mg daily conjugated equine oestrogens
2.0 mg daily oestradiol
1.5 mg daily piperazine oestrone sulphate
2.5 mg daily tibolone

Patch   50 µg oestradiol patches twice a week

Gel   2 'blobs' daily, each containing 0.75 mg oestradiol (Oestrogel)

Note: not all HRT products are licensed for the prevention of osteoporosis; if in doubt, ask the prescribing doctor.

women. Nevertheless, long-term use of the Pill for this purpose is not advised, partly because it does not provide continuous oestrogen and partly because of the additional risk of thrombosis associated with synthetic oestrogens.

The dose listed on the packet is likely to be given in milligrams (mg), rather than the smaller microgram (µg or mcg) doses found in non-oral HRT. Tablets contain more oestrogen because much of an oral dose is demolished by the gut and liver (see Chapter 4). Women who want to ensure that they are receiving an adequate dose to prevent osteoporosis can cross-check with the guidelines in Figure 10.1 for post-menopausal women of any age. Younger women who lack hormones may need a higher dose than those given to prevent menopausal symptoms. Only a few tablet brands come in such doses.

Some women have particular problems with side-effects when they take HRT by mouth. For example, oestrogen tablets can cause nausea, although this often disappears as the body adjusts. Other gastrointestinal side-effects may be more persistent. Usually these can be avoided by taking oestrogen in a different way, e.g. through the skin.

Many women find tablets are familiar and convenient. Although they must be remembered daily, they can be popped into a handbag just in case. But such a frequent routine doesn't suit everybody. Some women prefer using a twice or once-a-week method, such as skin patches. Others dislike taking tablets because they are a constant reminder of being medicated or of their condition (see Sherri, Chapter 6).

Oestrogen Skin Patches

One of the advertisements promoting HRT patches to doctors shows a transparent plastic circle in the dimple of a woman's shapely buttock. The reality is a lot less glamorous. For a start, anyone as young as the woman in the ad will probably need a larger patch, perhaps two. Also, like ordinary skin plasters, HRT patches tend to look their best before they get creased with wear and go grey round the edges. At least, patches are less likely to fall off in the bath, shower or pool.

The early skin patches were made of fairly thick plastic. This protected the central fluid bubble that contained oestradiol dissolved in alcohol. These 'reservoir' patches have been overtaken by 'matrix' patches, which are thinner because the hormone is laced into the adhesive (e.g. Fematrix). Matrix patches are more elegant, but they have lost the advantage of being re-usable should they come off.

Oestradiol is absorbed from the underside of the patch through the skin and subcutaneous fat into the bloodstream. Although some of it is converted into oestrone, most of it remains as oestradiol. This partial conversion is notable for two reasons. Firstly, it means that GPs can check the effect of patches using the standard 'oestrogen' blood test (although this is not usually necessary and women's results can be very variable). Secondly, it leads to an oestradiol:oestrone ratio similar to that found in pre-menopausal women. Doctors describe patches as 'more physiological' (body-like) for this reason. The gradual way in which patches release hormone is also seen as more physiological than, say, the daily wave produced by a tablet. These aspects of patches sound comforting, although those who question the use of HRT would argue that there is nothing 'body-like' about introducing hormones from an outside source after the menopause.

Patches may be changed once or twice weekly depending on the brand. Sometimes women have to apply a new patch early, perhaps because the previous one fell off or they prefer to swim without one. Women can worry that doing so will increase their dose. However, a fresh patch is not 'stronger'. Patches release hormone steadily until they run out, so the only way of increasing the dose is to provide more skin contact by using a larger patch or several patches at once.

At present the following sizes/doses are available: 25, 40, 50, 75, 80 or 100 µg. In-between or higher doses can be created by wearing two different sizes. Women in the natural menopause often use 50 µg, but younger women who lack hormones may need 100 µg or more. Girls who need small doses of HRT for puberty (see Chapter 6) may be advised to cut up a 25 µg matrix patch.

Patient information leaflets recommend placing the patch on clean dry unbroken skin below the waist. However, some positions are more practical than others. A patch under the waistband can rub. If it is put on sensitive skin near the pubic area, it may be painful to remove. The buttocks are a good position, but it may take a bit of practice to find out where to place the patch so that it won't catch on underwear, tights or the toilet seat.

Women can find that the skin under the patch becomes irritated. The alcohol contained in reservoir patches was often the culprit. Matrix patches avoid this problem and the adhesive is less likely to cause allergy, but the covered skin can still develop a reaction. Sometimes the irritation can be relieved by removing the patch early and starting a new one (since matrix patches aren't reusable) on a fresh area. It also helps to avoid talc, perfume and lotions. However, reactions can build up and some women have to rest their skin by using another type of HRT for a while or altogether.

Women can worry about wearing a patch under a bikini, in communal showers or changing rooms or in front of their lovers. These worries can be resolved by abandoning a patch for several hours.

Usually this can be done without ill effects (apart from wasting a patch) as menopausal symptoms take time to set in.

Patches often leave a grey rim of adhesive, which is difficult to remove. Rubbing the marks with baby oil can help. Alternatively one can ask a pharmacist about wipes designed for patients who have to wear bandages regularly and need to remove adhesive quickly and easily. The wipes are not cheap, but they work.

Women may have practical reasons for choosing a type of HRT, but often the decision is emotional too. Sometimes women prefer the idea of the natural oestrogen in patches or simply feel less 'medicated' because they don't have to remember tablets. Younger women who have been obliged to take HRT describe liking patches because they felt able to put 'their problems behind them'.

Oestrogen Gel

Patches aren't the only way of applying oestradiol to the skin. Gel is the most popular form of HRT in France, where it has been used for many years. It is available to other European women, although only one brand has been available in the UK until recently.

This type of HRT may come in a canister that produces measured 'blobs' of a colourless gel (e.g. Oestrogel). The canister is easy to use and looks like many of the containers one might find in a bathroom cabinet, although it fits less readily into a handbag. Alternatively gel may come in sachets (e.g. Sandrena). A 'blob' of Oestrogel contains 0.75 mg of oestradiol. Women in the natural menopause are prescribed two measures daily (a dose equivalent to a 50 µg patch). Younger women who lack hormones may be advised to use more.

The gel is rubbed into the underside of the upper arms or legs or lower body. It takes five minutes to dry. The area must not be washed or have other lotions applied to it for an hour. The size of the area to be coated is specified (a template is provided) to help ensure correct absorption. Skin irritation is unlikely compared to patches because the skin is not enclosed and there is no adhesive. However, absorption is less controlled. The amount of oestradiol reaching the bloodstream can be affected by how widely the gel is applied, how well it is rubbed in and how much comes off on clothing.

Some women like using gel because they can fit it into a daily bath-room routine and there is no need to fiddle with or hide patches. Others find that having to cover a specified area and wait for the gel to dry before getting dressed is inconvenient. Using it before going to bed might seem like the obvious solution, but this can be awkward for women with partners as skin contact should be avoided for an hour after applying the gel to prevent it being absorbed by anyone else!

Oestrogen Implants

Implants are small dissolvable pellets that are injected under the skin of the lower abdomen. They can also be placed in a surgical wound and women often receive their first one during a hysterectomy and/or bilateral oophorectomy. Women with AIS may be given an implant after their gonadectomy. These pellets release small amounts of oes-tradiol into the bloodstream over the following months. This means women can forget about their HRT until a new implant is due. In the past women had to return to a hospital clinic for this service. Now it is offered by a variety of NHS and private menopause clinics and some family doctors.

The everyday convenience of implants has a lot of practical appeal. Furthermore, like patches, implants are said to be more 'physiological' because they release natural oestradiol slowly into the bloodstream and result in a favourable oestradiol:oestrone ratio. Since implants release oestradiol, their effect on blood levels can be monitored using the standard 'oestrogen' blood test if necessary, although the results can be variable and may be affected by body weight.[2]

However, implants do have disadvantages. For a start, they cannot be removed easily if problems or side-effects occur. By the same token, it is difficult to reduce the dose or change to another type of HRT. Also, implants can go on producing oestrogen for much longer than was thought originally. This means that a woman who wishes to stop HRT may find that she cannot avoid this lingering effect. This also explains why implants have become associated with a problem known as tachyphylaxis. This term is used when women get less and less relief from menopausal symptoms in spite of receiving more and more HRT. There seem to be two reasons why this problem has arisen with implants. One is to do with the implants themselves. The other is to do with the way some women react to them.

An implant is supposed to provide oestradiol for six months, then a new one is inserted. Usually a 50 mg implant produces a blood oestradiol level within the range found during the menstrual cycle. For example, a woman who has been on 50 mg implants for a year tends to have a blood level of about 400 pmol/L.[3] However, an implant can go on releasing oestradiol for much longer than six months; often two years or more. This means that a new implant can add to the lingering effect of a previous implant. Six months later another implant can add to this again and so on.

Perhaps it is easiest to imagine this effect as a graph that looks like an increasingly wobbly staircase. Each new implant creates another step up in hormone levels, but the higher the levels become, the sooner and more sharply they drop. These 'drops' may be what causes the feeling in some women that their implant is 'running out', although their next implant is not due. They may even get hot flushes. This can lead a woman to request a new implant and her doctor to give it. However, this may just add to the lingering effects of previous implants and create higher and even more wobbly hormone levels. The result can be that the patient experiences less and less relief even though her oestradiol levels continue to rise overall (tachyphylaxis). In some cases, women have suffered hot flushes although their oestradiol levels were above those found during the menstrual cycle, i.e. more than 1000 pmol/L. Doctors call this a 'supra-physiological' level (more than body-like).

The solution to this cumulative effect and the risk of tachyphylaxis may seem obvious: remove the previous implant before inserting a new one. Unfortunately finding and removing an old implant is rather like looking for a needle in a haystack. In which case, one might say, why renew women's implants every six months if they have not run out? This is a good question. In the past implants were inserted routinely without investigating a woman's blood levels. Indeed, as described above, doctors gave women *early* implants if their symptoms returned before the next one was due. In some cases, but not all, this set the stage for tachyphylaxis.

Some researchers have described tachyphylaxis as a form of 'oestrogen dependence' or even addiction because the body appears to need higher and higher doses to prevent the return of 'menopausal' symptoms.[4] These symptoms have been likened to withdrawal symptoms. However, doctors disagree about this interpretation. For example, opponents argue that there is no evidence that high oestrogen levels are dangerous.[5] They note that high levels tend to be seen as dangerous simply because they are high. Other doctors suggest that tachyphylaxis has more to do with some women's psychological problems than hormonal dips.[6]

None the less, doctors tend to be more cautious about the use of implants nowadays. Prescribing guidelines advise that implants should only be replaced after checking blood oestradiol levels and one research clinic recommends that 50 mg implants should be renewed only when symptoms return and blood levels are less than 400 pmol/L.[7] Others suggest that tachyphylaxis is less likely with 25 mg implants. However, some doctors disagree about the need for caution, arguing that implants produce better bone protection.[8] Tachyphylaxis has been recognized with implants, but it may be possible with other forms of HRT.

Combined HRT

Combined HRT is the term used for HRT that contains forms of oestrogen *and* progesterone. Usually a synthetic form of progesterone is used, i.e. a progestogen (progest*in* in USA). In Britain it is common practice to give progestogens to women with a uterus to protect them against the increased risk of endometrial cancer associated with unopposed oestrogen. Practice differs in the USA, where such women are given oestrogen-only HRT and monitored for pre-cancerous warning signs in the lining of the womb.

Usually combined HRT involves taking a form of oestrogen continuously and a progestogen for 10–14 days of every month. When the progestogen is finished and levels fall, the lining of the womb is shed as a 'period', or what doctors call a 'withdrawal bleed'. The amount of blood lost varies and some women may have very little or none at all. Doctors do not regard this as a problem as long as women take all their progestogen to prevent overstimulation of the lining by oestrogen.[9] This protection is important even if women hardly bleed.

Sometimes women are tempted to miss the progestogen because of side-effects, such as acne, headaches, bloating and symptoms like premenstrual tension. One family of progestogens, the C19 family, has a particular reputation for these side-effects (see Figure 4.3, page 65). For example, norethisterone, norgestrel and levonorgestrel are well known for causing problems. Women may find that it helps to switch to a member of the C21 family, such as dydrogesterone or medroxyprogesterone acetate. (Some women may read this and wonder why their doctor hasn't suggested switching. This may be because HRT brands containing C21 progestogens are relatively new.)

Side-effects may also be lessened by using a brand of HRT or the Pill with a lower dose of progestogen. However, the dose must be high enough to protect the lining of the womb from overstimulation by the accompanying oestrogen, otherwise the imbalance can lead eventually to endometrial cancer. Doctors have guidelines on the lowest doses of progestogen that can be used safely with standard doses of oestrogen.

Combined-HRT tablets can come in handy calendar packs not unlike those for the contraceptive pill (e.g. Prempak-C, Cyclo-Progynova, Femoston, Climagest, Nuvelle, Trisequens, etc.). Alternatively some brands have different forms for each hormone, perhaps an oestradiol skin patch with progestogen tablets (e.g. Evorel-Pak or

Femapack). For those who want to avoid tablets entirely or who want to try and reduce side-effects, combination skin patches are available now (e.g. Nuvelle TS, Estracombi). Here, oestradiol patches are used for two weeks, then combined patches for the following two weeks. Some women find that the dumb-bell-shaped combined patch is rather large, but this drawback may be minor for those who find non-oral progestogen causes fewer side-effects.

Oestrogen implants combined with a separate form of progestogen, perhaps tablets, are also an option. However, in this case women must continue taking a progestogen for as much as two years after the last implant to counteract any lingering effects.

Continuous Combined HRT

As its name suggests, this HRT involves taking *both* hormones every day without breaks. Since there are no gaps in medication, progestogen levels never fall enough to produce a 'period' – at least, in theory.

This might seem an odd, even worrying, idea. After all, wasn't progestogen added to HRT so that women would have regular withdrawal bleeds? Wasn't this regular shedding of the lining of the womb meant to reduce the risk of endometrial cancer associated with using oestrogen-only HRT? According to researchers, it is the balancing effect of progestogen that reduces this risk rather than the actual shedding of the lining.[10] Therefore forms of HRT have been developed that provide continuous progestogen and skip the need for regular bleeds. It is believed that these may prove popular with post-menopausal women who do not want the bother of 'periods'. They can also be convenient for women who lack mobility.

Continuous combined HRT also aims to simplify life by skipping the on/off pattern of medication. Several brands provide a single daily tablet containing both hormones (e.g. Premique, Kliofem, Climesse). Continuous HRT is also available as skin patches (e.g. Evorelconti). Although these brands can be described as 'bleed-free therapy', this may not be the case. For example, some women get irregular bleeding for the first 6–12 months as their bodies adjust to the continuous combination of hormones. This may be nothing more than annoying. However, sometimes women develop significant bleeding because the lining of the womb has grown more than expected and finally comes away. This can lead to a situation where doctors are obliged to clear out the lining just in case there are unwanted changes (endometrial hyperplasia, which can warn of endometrial cancer). Women may find themselves having an unexpected D&C as a result (see Denise, Chapter 3).

In general, doctors are advised not to prescribe continuous combined HRT until at least a year after a woman has had her last period.[11] Spotting or bleeding can be a persistent problem for younger women, who may be better off taking combined HRT and having regular withdrawal bleeds.[12] Sometimes spotting in older women can be prevented by altering the type and dose of progestogen. Since there are only a few brands of continuous HRT to choose from, doctors may prescribe separate brands of oestrogen and progestogen. This could mean taking two daily tablets or using patches alongside tablets. However, if irregular bleeding continues, women may have to take combined HRT in the usual way or reconsider taking HRT. Whatever its exact form, continuous combined HRT is still rather experimental treatment and little is known about its long-term use compared to more conventional forms of HRT (which also remain the subject of research).

A potential compromise is to use a brand of continuous HRT that allows a withdrawal bleed every three months (e.g. Tridestra). Here, oestradiol is taken for 70 days, then a combination of hormones is taken for 14 days. This is followed by seven days of an inactive tablet, which allows the hormone levels to fall. The lining of the womb is shed during this time. Again, this HRT is fairly new and experimental.

Tibolone

Tibolone (Livial) is an older drug that can be prescribed as continuous HRT to prevent menopausal symptoms and osteoporosis. Its ability to prevent heart disease is less clear. It is a synthetic compound that acts on oestrogen and progesterone receptors, but without stimulating the lining of the womb. This means it can be used by women who want to take HRT without having periods (see Bungy, Chapter 1). However, like the newer forms of continuous HRT described above, it can cause irregular bleeding if used less than 12 months after the last period. Younger women who need HRT may also develop spotting. It is not contraceptive.

Tibolone may be an option for women who suspect their endometriosis has returned in spite of having their ovaries removed at hysterectomy. Endometriosis is misplaced tissue like the lining of the womb, so the fact that tibolone doesn't stimulate the endometrium suggests it won't stimulate endometriosis either (recurrence occurs in response to oestrogen-only HRT in up to 5 per cent of cases.)[13]

Tibolone comes in one form: a 2.5 mg daily tablet. It has been suggested that tibolone may help women's libido more than conventional types of HRT because it acts on receptors for the androgen family of hormones (which includes testosterone). Some of its possible side-effects, such as acne and increases in facial hair, may also be explained by its effect on androgen receptors.

Testosterone

Testosterone therapy can be advised to restore libido. It is still experimental, as only a few placebo-controlled trials have been done.[14] Studies suggest that women who've had their ovaries removed may be most likely to benefit (and by implication, women born without functioning ovaries).

Testosterone therapy can be rather hit-and-miss as doctors try to lower the dose appropriately for women using products designed for men (although new brands are being developed). For example, Australian researchers recommend that doctors divide a 100 mg testosterone implant under sterile conditions to get a 50 mg dose.[15] Similarly in the USA 2.5 mg and 1.25 mg methyltestosterone tablets are available, but they may need to be divided with a pill-splitter to get a physiological dose (see Juanita, Chapter 6).

Whether the dose should be pharmacological or physiological is still a matter of debate. The few controlled studies that suggest that testosterone HRT may improve sexual arousal after oophorectomy have been criticized because they relied on pharmacological doses (i.e. higher than those produced by the body). Pre-menopausal blood levels of testosterone are about 50 ng/dL,[16] but women had levels of 111–133 ng/dL in one study and over 200 ng/dL in another. Pharmacological doses are more likely to cause side-effects such as acne, increased facial hair, altered liver function and occasional voice deepening (which may be irreversible).

The risk of side-effects can be reduced by reducing the dose.[17] An American doctor has argued that much lower, physiological doses (0.25–0.8 mg/day of methyltestosterone) can produce beneficial effects on libido.[18] She also suggests that women have a sensitive 'window', i.e. a dose that works best for them but which may change as they age. These observations are based on her clinical experience with patients. At present there are no placebo-controlled studies of such low doses.

The risk of side-effects can also be reduced by choosing certain forms of therapy. For example, one researcher has noted that some side-effects, such as hair growth, are less likely when women use non-oral methods.[19] Implants use natural testosterone, but they can produce quite erratic pharmacological blood levels and may have a lingering effect that is difficult to alter if there are side-effects.[20] Early testing on testosterone skin patches for women suggests that they may have several advantages because they use natural testosterone and produce physiological levels.[21] Other doctors comment that testosterone HRT should be used only for the time it takes to restore libido in order to reduce the risk of side-effects.

In the UK implants are the only readily available form of testosterone HRT for women at the time of writing. Women may find that testosterone helps their libido, although individual reports (of rather different doses) vary (see Jane, Chapter 1 and Juanita, Chapter 6). If so, women may wish to discuss their doctor's views on the appropriate dose, the length of treatment and plans for monitoring their progress. The long-term risks and benefits of testosterone are not known.

Vaginal Oestrogen

All the types of HRT described so far are 'systemic' drugs, i.e. they affect the whole body 'system' and are meant to relieve menopausal problems. However, they do not solve the problem of vaginal dryness in some women. Alternatively women may not wish to take systemic HRT simply for vaginal dryness. In either case, their GP may suggest vaginal oestrogen (see Maureen, Chapter 3).

Vaginal oestrogen can be inserted as pessaries, smaller tablets or cream. An oestrogen-releasing vaginal ring (Estring) is also available in Europe. These products are designed to work on the surrounding tissues and therefore contain lower doses of oestrogen than other forms of HRT. However, it can be misleading to assume that they won't affect the rest of the body. As the use of patches and gels shows, oestrogen is absorbed through bodily surfaces, and the vaginal walls are no exception. However, this depends on the state of the lining. Once the lining becomes less dry, oestrogen is more likely to reach the bloodstream.

The amount of systemic absorption can be reduced by using the vaginal ring or a brand containing natural rather than synthetic oestrogens.[22] The following products contain natural oestrogens: Vagifem tablets, Ovestin cream and Ortho-Gynest cream/pessaries. Premarin cream contains conjugated equine oestrogens (see page 61). Ortho-Dienoestrol cream and Tampovagan pessaries use the synthetic dienoestrol and stilboestrol respectively.

Usually the instructions with cream or pessaries advise frequent use to begin with, followed by a prompt reduction. This is partly because oestrogen is absorbed more rapidly once the vaginal lining has been primed. Also, the lining appears to become less sensitive if vaginal oestrogen is overused. Researchers suggest that women stop using the product for a while if this happens and then retry using a lower dose to maintain sensitivity.[23] In any event, vaginal creams are not intended to be used indefinitely, especially in women who have not had a hysterectomy. Premarin cream may be prescribed for long-term use if a progestogen is taken for 10–14 days each cycle to oppose the effects of oestrogen on the lining of the womb.

The vaginal ring can be inserted at home and will fit women whether they have a cervix or not. It is designed to stay in place for three months and slowly release oestradiol before being renewed. Current guidelines are that vaginal rings should not be used for more than two years.

Vaginal oestrogen can also help cystitis,[24] which can be more common in women with low hormones (although it has not been found to help stress incontinence). Women with AIS have found that bouts of cystitis that occur in spite of taking systemic HRT can be cured by vaginal oestrogen.

Vaginal dryness and cystitis may also improve with non-hormonal products (e.g. Aci-jel, Senselle), which increase the acidity of the vagina, thereby maintaining a defence against bacteria. Replens and KY jelly only act as lubricants. Alternatives which may help include pelvic floor exercises, dietary changes and Vitamin E.

Some vaginal products can damage latex (this includes some non-hormonal preparations), so women using condoms are advised to check the instructions. Women are also warned not to use vaginal oestrogen creams as lubricants during sex because the hormone can be absorbed by their partner.

Women who lack vaginal length report that vaginal oestrogen helps the use of dilators.

Follow-up Care

At present, in the UK, there are no national guidelines on monitoring for women on HRT. Nor is it clear where the responsibility for follow-up care should lie or what form it should take. Women can be on HRT for many different reasons. In most cases, they will be healthy women who are taking HRT to prevent menopausal symptoms or longer-term problems and their care simply falls under their GP. Alternatively women can begin HRT as part of treatment in a range of clinics, e.g. gynaecology, endocrinology, oncology, adolescent services. When they leave, their follow-up care falls to their GP. Sometimes women may find or be referred to a specialist menopause clinic (see More Help), although often this is a regional or private service.

GPs and their staff may well be best placed to monitor women on HRT since they are local, accessible and have an ongoing overview. However, GPs can have difficulty building up enough relevant experience, even if HRT interests them. Most GPs have about 2000 patients and only a small proportion will be women on HRT. Of these, perhaps two or three will be women who need HRT from an early age. Furthermore, the range of hormone treatment is such that GPs are unlikely to be familiar with women's reactions to all types.

A 'shared-care' approach has been put forward by the Royal College of Obstetricians and Gynaecologists, Royal College of General Practitioners and National Osteoporosis Society. This urges hospital and community staff to work together to ensure, among other things, 'regular monitoring' of women who have an early hysterectomy and go on to or subsequently need HRT. It is less clear what this will mean in reality. Some doctors have suggested that care be shared between a relevant specialist and the GP as it is, for example, while women are pregnant. Alternatively national guidelines for the follow-up care of women on HRT could be produced, as they have been for the care of women on the contraceptive pill or groups such as diabetics. However, these would need to be informed by research. At present, it is not clear what monitoring should be done.

In the meantime, the only option available to most women hoping for appropriate follow-up care is to find a GP who is interested in HRT. At least, they are more likely to have experience of patients' problems with treatment and to be willing to keep up with developments. Some GP surgeries have computerized systems for repeat prescriptions and invite patients for an annual check-up before they can renew their HRT. Other practices do not have a recall system and women visit if they have any problems.

The check-up may be an ordinary appointment with the GP or nurse practitioner. It may be part of a well-woman or menopause clinic run by the surgery. Either way, it is mainly an opportunity to talk about any difficulties with the prescription, in which case a different type or dose of HRT may be suggested. Usually this is done without doing hormone tests. This can seem surprising; however, blood tests may not pick up the effects of HRT (see Chapter 4). Even when they do, the results vary so much that test results may not be a guide to a treatment's effectiveness. So doctors rely on how women feel in themselves and their symptoms or side-effects.

During the check-up, women are likely to have their blood pressure taken and may have a breast examination. The visit may also be used as an opportunity to do well-woman tests that are due, such as a smear, or give lifestyle advice. Other tests may be done in response to individual problems.

Many women on HRT have questions about breast screening. In the UK mammograms are done as part of the NHS National Breast Screening Programme. Women aged 50–64 are automatically invited for this test every three years, whether or not they are on HRT. The age group and three-year interval were defined on the basis of research. This suggested who should be screened, and how often, to ensure that more good was done (e.g. by detecting breast cancer early) than harm (e.g. by worrying women unnecessarily because of false positive results).

Women over 65 are entitled to request regular mammograms and some medical authors suggest that they probably should if they are on HRT.[25] As explained in Chapter 5, this option is not available to younger women, although any woman with problems that need investigation, such as a breast lump, will get immediate referral. At present, doctors are not clear whether younger women should have mammograms before beginning HRT treatment.

Given the publicity for osteoporosis, women may also ask about bone scans. Here the position is rather different. There is no *national* screening programme, and research suggests that this would not be an effective way to tackle osteoporosis. Instead, women in high-risk groups (see Figure 5.6, p. 92) are eligible (but not specifically invited) for five-yearly DXA bone scans on the NHS. This emphasis on high-risk groups may explain why some women find that their doctor is not willing to refer them. However, even women who fall into these categories can find that their GP is reluctant. In this case, the doctor may consider that there is no medical reason to gain further information for the woman who is on HRT, i.e. who is already on the recommended treatment. Equally, if a woman has already refused HRT, then the GP may see little point in a scan unless it is likely to change her mind.

An annual HRT check-up can be a welcome opportunity to discuss these questions or an irritation if it means taking time off work or a busy home schedule just to get one's prescription renewed. However, given some of the uncertainties about HRT, women who have been prescribed long-term treatment can find regular follow-up care reassuring. Women who do not receive check-ups may be quite happy to visit the surgery as and when they need to; others can feel very adrift.

Stopping HRT

The length of time women are advised to stay on HRT will depend on their reasons for being on it in the first place and the balance of risks and benefits in their case. Women who begin HRT mid-life as treatment for menopausal symptoms may want to reconsider after about 5–10 years given the extra risk of breast cancer (see Figure 5.7,

p. 96). However, the risk:benefit equation is rather different for women who lack hormones at an early age (see page 95). Usually they are advised to take HRT until they are 50 or 60 years old.

Women who want to stop HRT can do so immediately, but this can be a very uncomfortable experience. Symptoms such as hot flushes may return with a vengeance, perhaps because of the sudden drop in blood hormone levels. Younger women on higher doses may have particular problems, presumably because the fall in levels is that much greater. That said, some women can stop HRT and have no symptoms at all.

In general, doctors advise women to come off HRT slowly to reduce the chances of menopausal symptoms returning, or their severity if they do. For women taking tablets, GPs may prescribe the lowest possible dose and suggest that they adjust to this for a month or so before reducing the dose further by halving the pills or taking them on alternate days. The exact regime will depend on the type of HRT. The gap between tablets can be increased until it is possible to stop altogether. Women on matrix patches can be given a smaller size/dose (the smallest is 25 μg) or advised to cut their existing patches into appropriate sections before following a similar pattern of reduction. Women on combined HRT are likely to have lighter withdrawal bleeds during the months of adjustment and a brief bleed may follow sometime after stopping medication.

Women who are on combined implant and progestogen therapy face a specific problem. They will need to continue taking a progestogen for some time, perhaps one to two years, after their last implant to counteract any ongoing stimulation of the womb lining. This remaining influence explains why women with ovarian failure can have apparently spontaneous 'periods' after implant therapy. In the past, this was mistaken for the return of a true menstrual cycle because the effects of implants were not fully understood (see Susan, Chapter 7).

Young women who give up HRT suddenly can be surprised by the severity of their menopausal symptoms, especially if they didn't suffer such problems before their diagnosis. It seems that women can only get symptoms such as hot flushes once their bodies have been sensitized by hormones, either those they produce at puberty or through the early use of HRT.

Coming off HRT slowly is the best way of reducing the chances of menopausal symptoms returning, but several other strategies may help. For example, if possible, it is advisable to stop when the weather is cooler since hot flushes have been related to core body temperature. Similarly it may be wise to choose a time when nothing special is planned that might be spoilt. Stressful periods at home or work may be more difficult to predict or avoid but, again, this may not be the best time since stress can make hot flushes worse and vice versa.

II

NATURAL PROGESTERONE

Natural progesterone is not new. What is new is the idea that it can be used alone as hormone replacement therapy, and the fierce debate that has developed. This chapter cannot resolve the controversy any more than those who are fully engaged in it seem able to at present. However, it can provide some background and look briefly at some of the arguments being used.

Why Progesterone?

The conventional medical view is that women become oestrogen deficient after the menopause because their oestrogen levels fall. This is thought to be serious because women will lack oestrogen for the next 30–40 years, rather longer than Nature intended. Prolonged oestrogen deficiency is said to increase women's risks of heart disease and osteoporosis and to be remedied by replacing the missing hormone: oestrogen.

Progestogens entered this picture when doctors realized that oestrogen replacement therapy led to an increase in endometrial cancer in women who had not had a hysterectomy. They discovered that adding progestogens (synthetic versions of progesterone) reduced this extra risk. These progestogens were introduced to control a potential side-effect of taking oestrogen, not because doctors saw menopausal women as progesterone deficient. So why are some doctors now taking the view that women can suffer progesterone deficiency and therefore benefit from using natural progesterone?

Understanding the arguments involves going back a few steps to what happens in the run-up to the menopause. At this stage women ovulate less frequently before stopping altogether. Since progesterone is the hormone released by the follicle-egg sac left behind at ovulation, this means that women also produce less and less progesterone. Oestrogen is released by active follicles whether one of them ovulates or not, so levels of this hormone do not fall in the same way during this time. Oestrogen only drops when the ovaries run out of egg follicles and the menstrual cycle comes to an end. Even then, women still produce some oestrogen from elsewhere. In contrast, their progesterone levels fall to almost nothing.

According to Dr Lee, the main advocate for natural progesterone, 'oestrogen dominance' occurs when a woman has too much oestrogen compared to progesterone.[1] Her oestrogen levels will be problematic, whether high or low, if they are not balanced by her progesterone. Taking this view, the relative lack of progesterone in the run-up to the menopause is not a natural state. Instead, it is the reason for symptoms of 'oestrogen dominance' during this time such as water retention, sweet cravings, weight gain, premenstrual depression, lack of libido, heavy or irregular periods, fibrocystic breasts and fibroids.[2] Here the mistake is not seen as Nature's, but 'ours' because the inadequate Western diet does not promote healthy follicles and regular ovulation. Furthermore, this diet cannot buffer the eventual hormonal changes. If one accepts this theory, then the idea of adding further oestrogen is misguided, if not laughable. Instead, as its supporters argue, the remedy is dietary changes and replacement of natural progesterone.

Natural progesterone is seen as the hormone that is genuinely missing. Replacing it will balance the unwanted effects of oestrogen dominance during the menopause. In addition, natural progesterone is thought to reverse – not just delay – osteoporosis.[3] Dr Lee highlights how bone loss begins during the decade of increasingly erratic ovulation (and therefore falling progesterone) in the run-up to the menopause and suggests that progesterone deficiency is a more logical explanation than oestrogen deficiency, which begins after the menopause. He also presents his conclusion that natural progesterone skin cream reversed osteoporosis among a series of his patients, increasing bone density by between 2.6 and 22.4 per cent over three years[4] as measured by a DPA machine (dual photon absorptiometry).

As its supporters stress frequently, natural progesterone treatment is unlike conventional HRT because it avoids oestrogen and contains progesterone, not progestogen. The progesterone is identical to that produced by the body and intended for use in physiological doses. The naturalness of the product and the dosage are put forward as reasons to assume its safety and explain its few side-effects.[5]

The Main Debates

Natural progesterone has many supporters among women and some among doctors. It also has many opponents, medical and non-medical. Ironically, despite its blend of medical and alternative ideas, the use of natural progesterone has been attacked from both sides.

Few doctors have been drawn by the theory of oestrogen dominance and serious doubts have been expressed about the validity of Dr Lee's findings that natural progesterone skin cream reverses osteoporosis. The results were greeted with scepticism since they were not from a randomized controlled trial that can exclude the placebo effect (see page 207) and other kinds of bias. Other complaints include the possible effects of other factors on the results, such as the dietary advice and the oestrogen women were also receiving in some cases, and the lack of detail in published accounts to enable an independent assessment.[6]

There is some acceptance of the view that progesterone may influence bone tissue. Bone loss has been found in women with menstrual cycles that have a short second half (when progesterone is produced). Doctors also acknowledge that bone has progesterone receptors and that laboratory experiments have shown that bone-replacing cells can be stimulated by progesterone.[7] However, this is not accepted as conclusive since 'in vitro' (test-tube) results are not always repeated when studied 'in vivo' (live) within the body. Doubts remain about whether progesterone can cause substantial gains in bone density that reverse osteoporosis and, in particular, whether this can be achieved using a skin cream which is said to deliver physiological doses.

This scepticism is partly because most treatments prevent bone loss, rather than adding bone. On current treatments, women's bone density often increases initially but then evens out, i.e. osteoporosis is stalled, not reversed. Another reason for doubt is that existing methods of delivering natural progesterone use other routes into the body (injections, vaginal and anal suppositories) and much higher doses. Therefore questions have converged on whether a skin cream could deliver progesterone and, if so, whether small amounts could have such an unexpected effect.

Unlike oestradiol, progesterone doesn't dissolve in alcohol and so the skin cream only became available when a method of dissolving natural progesterone in Vitamin E was patented. Having patented the delivery system, there was nothing to be lost by using the natural hormone rather than an altered version. However, the product was not envisaged as HRT. Instead, it was sold in the USA as a moisturizing cream (a situation that is becoming more tightly regulated) until it attracted the attention of Dr Lee, who used it among his patients.

An early criticism of the cream used as HRT was that it did no more than accumulate in the skin. The reply was that only unimportant ingredients, such as waxes, remain in the skin and the cream's effectiveness should not be reduced if women follow the advice to apply it to a new site on each occasion.[8] Dr Lee has also said that the progesterone can be 'lost' in the fat cells for the first few months of use if menopausal women are very progesterone deficient.[9]

More recently a medical paper reported a small double-blind placebo-controlled trial of Pro-Gest™ (the product cited by Dr Lee). The researchers found that the cream led to very low levels of progesterone in the bloodstream, even though women used 2–4 times the recommended dose.[10] This led them to conclude that it could not protect the lining of the womb adequately if used as part of combined HRT and could not save bone. They also commented that a 2 oz jar of cream contained only 200 mg of progesterone.

According to supporters, such findings can be questioned on several grounds. For example, they say that 200 mg of progesterone is atypical for Pro-Gest™ and women's absorption should have been measured using salivary tests because they are more sensitive.[11] The progesterone content of the sampled cream is problematic (see also Figure 11.1) and one is left to decide why quality-control systems for the marketing company on the one hand, and the researchers on the other, came up with such different results and whether this was because the contents were tested using different systems, as supporters suggest.

Salivary tests are a more sensitive measure of progesterone.[12] However, doctors say that progesterone levels are lower in saliva than blood, therefore salivary tests need to be more sensitive, i.e. able to pick up such low levels. It follows that if women in the study had low blood levels of progesterone after using the cream, their salivary levels would be lower still (although measurable with the sensitive salivary test). Yet supporters argue that, unlike other delivery methods, progesterone cream leads to *higher* levels in saliva than in blood. They add that the proportion of 'biological available' hormone (not bound to protein) is greater in saliva. The latter is true, but doctors and biochemists find it difficult to agree that progesterone cream is a misunderstood exception because they cannot see any sensible explanation for the view that skin cream leads to higher progesterone levels in saliva than in the body's circulation.

Arguments about natural progesterone cream come from other quarters as well. Those who question the need for women to use hormones see no reason to regard natural progesterone as a special case either. As one alternative practitioner has commented, the menopause is a time when it is natural for the body to stop producing progesterone, so how can it be natural to replace it?[13] Dietary improvements will ease the menopause by enabling women to balance their own hormones – not another version of hormone replacement therapy. Others have argued that there are dangers in seeing natural progesterone in the same light as a vitamin supplement.[14] Women are also warned about embracing progesterone too quickly given the history of oestrogen, which was used as HRT before its relationship with

Figure 11.1 Progesterone and wild yams

- progesterone is not found in wild yam or other plants (e.g. soy)
- a substance with a related chemical structure called diosgenin is

- laboratories turn diosgenin from yams (or soy) into synthetic progestogens
- they also turn diosgenin into natural progesterone
- the body does not have enzymes that can perform the same conversion

- no one has shown that the body turns diosgenin from wild yam into progesterone
- wild yam can affect the body (see Chapter 12), but not because the body converts yam diosgenin into progesterone

- some products contain extract of wild yam
- some contain progesterone described as 'extract of wild yam'
- some contain wild yam described as a chemical precursor of progesterone

- progesterone is a *laboratory* extract of wild yam; so are synthetic progestogens
- wild yam is only a *chemical* precursor of progesterone in the sense that it can be converted in a laboratory (not the body)

Dr Lee advises a cream that provides 400–500 mg of natural progesterone per ounce; others may contain too much or too little.[15] He also warns against products that use mineral oil and other imitators where the progesterone is not in an appropriate cream with the result that gradually it becomes worthless on exposure to air in the jar.

endometrial cancer was understood and, some would argue, is still being used without adequate knowledge of its risks.

Concern has also been expressed about the 'naturalness' of natural progesterone, especially since this label offers reassurance and implies safety. After all, natural progesterone is synthesized in a laboratory before it is added to the cream.[16] Advocates reply that even the body 'synthesizes' and that, in this case, the laboratory and bodily processes yield exactly the same molecule (unlike synthetic progestogens, which cannot be produced by the body).[17] They emphasize that the dosage does not exceed 'Nature's own recommendation', i.e. the 20–30 mg/day that the ovary produces after ovulation. This dosage sounds reassuring until one remembers that the ovaries stop producing progesterone after the menopause.[18]

The wisdom of using natural progesterone alongside oestrogen therapy has also been questioned, given the need to protect women from the increased risk of endometrial cancer associated with taking inadequately opposed oestrogen. Doctors who advocate natural progesterone recommend that women halve their oestrogen dose before using natural progesterone in this way.[19] Other doctors point to the lack of data about the safety of doing this when it is not clear what dose of natural progesterone is protective.[20] However, in general, advocates see no need for women to take oestrogen at all, except in the few cases where symptoms such as hot flushes and vaginal dryness do not improve after several months of natural progesterone treatment.

Since the initial interest in natural progesterone, the waters have been muddied further because several progesterone creams have appeared on the market as well as creams that contain extracts of wild yam. Now the situation is such that certain progesterone creams are promoted as 'extracts of wild yam', some wild yam creams make a point of containing 'a chemical precursor of progesterone' and others emphasize that they are 'hormone-free' (see Figure 11.1). Satisfied customers are presented by all sides, as indeed they are for the original natural progesterone cream and, indirectly, for conventional HRT.

Conventional HRT is promoted on the basis of extensive (if not conclusive) research. Similar resources have not been committed to natural progesterone. This may be due to vested interests. It may be because transdermal (skin) methods of HRT have advanced only recently. It may be because a natural progesterone skin cream that delivers physiological doses lacks credibility. In the meantime, drug companies have increased the range of patented methods for delivering natural progesterone (in the higher doses), e.g. micronized progesterone tablets and a vaginal gel (Crinone). Doctors have also pointed out that women can choose HRT containing dydrogesterone, a well-established progestogen, which is converted rapidly by the body into natural progesterone.

Using Natural Progesterone

Up-to-date information on how to obtain and use an appropriate product is available elsewhere (see page 278). Conventional methods of using natural progesterone, which have been available on the NHS for some time, are not advised by Dr Lee as hormone replacement because the doses are too high. However, goods containing progesterone cannot be offered over the counter or by mail order in the UK and it is illegal to supply such products without a prescription from within the country. Some doctors will prescribe the recommended natural progesterone treatment as part of a private consultation or on a private prescription.

Although most well-known as a skin cream, natural progesterone also comes as an oil, capsule or drops to be held under the tongue. Dr Lee advises women to apply the cream or oil to areas where the skin is thin and blushes easily, such as the neck, upper chest, inner arms and thighs and to rotate the sites. The drops and capsules are seen as less desirable because the hormone is absorbed and cleared out of the body so rapidly that there is quite a hormonal swing. Since the capsules enter the body via the stomach, they contain much higher doses to compensate for the fact that the liver is quick to dismantle natural progesterone. Such high doses may cause drowsiness. The dosage and pattern of use depend on the symptoms being treated. Incorrect use can lead to spotting in women who still have a menstrual cycle.

Postscript

Women's interest in natural progesterone is understandable. As a recent editorial on alternative medicine has commented, today people are suspicious of drug-company profits and many conventional therapies have unwanted risks or side-effects. Also, people want a say in what treatments get developed and tested. Natural progesterone cream appears to offer an easy effective option that meets women's needs while bypassing the profit motive and conventional medical wisdom. To many women, that sounds appealing and worth a try. If it works, they may not care whether it is the placebo effect or not. Yet this is not without costs, the profit motive or its disreputable side, as the proliferation of skin creams has shown.

At present, the arguments about natural progesterone look set to continue until further studies are done, perhaps even thereafter. Meanwhile, natural progesterone has become more widely available and in that sense women's choices may have improved. For those against the use of hormones, this extra choice will miss the point and be like watching women switch to unleaded petrol rather than opting to protect the environment by not using the car. Others will welcome the way that natural progesterone has been made available to women and pay tribute to consumer power. In time they may be able to say that the campaign was on a par with the patient lobbying that gave AIDS sufferers access to the drug AZT before clinical testing had been completed – a drug that turned out to be beneficial. However, treatments that have been passionately advocated, even genuinely, by a few high-profile health professionals and tested in response to subsequent public demand are not new and many have proved to be a waste of money.[21]

In short, natural progesterone could go down in history as a (doctor-led?) women's revolution that challenged the multinational drug companies and research establishments[22] or it could become as infamous as the Di Bella cancer treatment, which led to public demonstrations in favour of government-funded testing in Italy, yet was shown to be ineffective.[23]

12

OTHER ALTERNATIVES

There are plenty of alternatives for women who want help with menopausal symptoms but do not want to take hormones (natural or otherwise). However, anyone who starts their search by walking into a health-food shop or local chemist could be forgiven for feeling rather dazed by the number of supplements aimed at them. Turning to mail-order suppliers listed in the back of health magazines or opening the phone book to look for an alternative practitioner can be equally daunting. Venture on to the Internet and it will be buzzing with information and products. How does one make sense of it all?

This chapter provides an initial guide to some of the advice that women are likely to come across. This ranges from dietary and herbal supplements to alternative therapies. Further information is suggested in More Help, including where to obtain lists of registered alternative practitioners.

Soy Foods

Soy is attracting a lot of attention as a way of preventing menopausal symptoms because it is an important part of the diet in Asian countries where such problems are rarely reported. Indeed, much is made of the fact that the Japanese language does not have a word for 'hot flushes'. Perhaps different cultural perceptions could explain this word's absence, but another possibility is that soy contains beneficial substances.

Researchers have found that soy contains high levels of isoflavones, an important group of phytoestrogens, i.e. substances in plants that have oestrogenic effects. They have also confirmed that phytoestrogens can be consumed in sufficient quantities to influence the body. Indeed, Japanese women, who eat 2–3 servings of soy a day (50–100 mg isoflavones) have 1000 times more phytoestrogen in their urine than their own oestrogen.[1]

The idea that this could be a good thing may seem curious because surely one wouldn't want oestrogenic substances to increase to such levels? However, phytoestrogens are much weaker than oestradiol, varying from 1/250th to 1/1000th of its strength, and are believed to be *selective*. This means they may act as 'skeleton keys' unlocking oestrogenic change in some cells and preventing it in others. Some researchers think that isoflavones could be like SERMs, the so-called 'designer' oestrogens.

As a result of this selective action, phytoestrogens may bring about changes in women that depend on their existing oestrogen levels. In pre-menopausal women, they may reduce the effects of oestradiol by competing with it and preventing its stronger action on the receptors. After the menopause, phytoestrogens may supplement women's falling levels and prevent troublesome symptoms. In other words, they may be anti-oestrogenic before the menopause, but oestrogenic afterwards.

Researchers are interested in finding out whether these theories are as good as they sound. Much work remains to be done, but it appears that 45 mg isoflavones/day can affect women's hormone levels and their menstrual cycles. It also lowers post-menopausal women's levels of FSH and LH. A recent review commented that 4 out of 5 studies found soy led to some improvement in hot flushes and 3 out of 5 reported oestrogenic changes in the vaginal lining.[2] There was a large placebo effect for hot flushes and often all benefits faded when the diet was stopped. One serving of soy foods, such as 56 g of tofu, provides 25–40 mg of isoflavones (mainly genistein and daidzein). Genistein has 1/250th of the strength of oestradiol and is one of the stronger phytoestrogens. However, the isoflavone content and its merits can vary quite widely for different soy foods (see Figure 12.1).

Figure 12.1 Quick guide to soy foods

Soy beans are available in traditional forms such as tofu, tempeh and miso, as well as newer products such as soya milks, breads and powders. Some forms of soy are richer in isoflavones than others, e.g. tofu contains 10 times more than soya milk. Fermented soy foods (e.g. tempeh) contain fewer isoflavones, but the body is able to make better use of them.

Soy beans can be bought tinned or dried (soak in water overnight). Pop them in a soup or casserole or roast them as a snack. Tofu is bean curd, although it is firm and silky compared to dairy curds. It can be cubed or minced and, given its bland taste, it is readily substituted in meat dishes or stir-fries. Some people prefer the fermented pressed soybean cake tempeh, which has a smoky flavour. Miso is a salty fermented paste that can be used to season soups, sauces and marinades.

Soya milks and desserts are also available (check the sugar content). Some people are happy with soya milk on breakfast cereals, others prefer to disguise the somewhat chalky taste by substituting it in a milkshake or using it in cooking. Try the vanilla dessert instead of cream or custard. Breads containing soy (and linseed) have come on to the market more recently. Soy flour can also be used for baking breads and fruit loaves; cooks advise substituting $\frac{1}{4}$ to $\frac{1}{3}$ of wheat flour to get a moist texture that is not too dense.

Some of these soy foods can be found in supermarkets (the milks tend to be with long-life dairy milks). Health-food shops also sell the milks and a range of other products, e.g. soy protein powder (the latter is often aimed at muscle builders and convalescents). Not all processed products retain their isoflavones, so check the label; if in doubt, choose a traditional food. 'Defatted' soy loses its ability to improve lipoprotein levels in ways that may reduce the risk of heart disease.[3] Soy supplements are available, but it is not clear whether these are preferable since research has looked at dietary soy.

Isoflavones are also found in chickpeas, although to a lesser extent. Humous (chick-pea pâté or dip) is available in supermarkets, as are tinned chick peas, which make a nutty addition to casseroles as well as potato or bean salads. Alfalfa contains the isoflavone daidzein.[4]

There are many other ways of using soy foods as easy alternatives or creative dishes in their own right. Anyone new to soy who wants to explore further will find recipe books full of helpful ideas, including how to get away with soy in family meals.

Soy has also attracted attention because Asian countries have much lower rates of heart disease and breast cancer than the West. It appears that a high consumption of soy can improve lipoproteins and dilate coronary arteries.[5] One study has reported a significant increase in bone density due to soy, which requires further investigation.[6] Some of these beneficial effects may be related to phytoestrogens, especially genistein. Others could be due to the essential fatty acids ('essential' to the diet) in soy, which enable prostaglandin metabolism. Prostaglandins are substances involved, for example, in the management of blood vessels, the stickiness of platelets in clotting and the inflammatory response. Soy is a good source of two important essential fatty acids: omega-3 series (also found in fish oils) and omega-6 series linolenic acid (also found with GLA in evening primrose oil). Prostaglandin pathways also require minerals such as calcium, zinc and magnesium.

Linseed (Flaxseed)

Linseed contains another important group of phytoestrogens, the lignans. Lignans are also found in many fibre-providing foods such as beans, wheat, rye, vegetables, fruit (especially plums, cherries and berries), bean sprouts, sunflower seeds, sesame seeds and nuts. However, linseed has an exceptionally high concentration of lignans and so a daily tablespoonful is an effective serving. One or two tablespoons can be added easily to breakfast cereals or used as a topping on yoghurt or fruit. Studies have found that linseed can reduce hot flushes and vaginal dryness, although for hot flushes there was also a large placebo effect.[7]

Linseed can be found in phytoestrogen breads (with soy) in supermarkets or bought as a loose product in health-food shops. It is also available as linseed oil capsules or a liquid supplement. Like soya, linseed is an important source of omega-3 essential fatty acids.

Herbal Remedies

Herbal remedies make use of plants with oestrogenic effects. For example, ingredients such as red clover, liquorice and glycine max produce oestrogenic changes in animals. Dandelion, used in traditional Chinese medicine, contains the phytoestrogen coumestrol and alfalfa contains daidzein. However, herbalists tend to see menopausal symptoms as signs of kidney, liver and blood disharmony rather than hormonal deficiencies. Thus herbal formulas for the menopause can include liquorice for anxiety and depression, dandelion to cleanse the liver and herbs to improve the circulation and cleanse the blood. The latter may be dong quai (tang kuei), paeonia, rehmannia, ginger, cinnamon, hoelen, pinellia, cnidium, persica and/or pueraria. Pueraria, a reputed aphrodisiac, has been found to contain a potent phytoestrogen, miroestrol.[8]

Other herbs that act like weak oestrogens include wild yam root, black cohosh and fennel seeds.[9] Some of these and Chinese herbs such as dong quai appear in menopause formulas and supplements for sale in chemists and health-food shops (see Figure 12.2). However, many herbalists advise brewing the herbs to extract the active ingredients rather than expecting the body to do this. Brewing can avoid some of the side-effects that may result from taking herbs as supplements.

Traditional recipes often advise several complementary plants, but a single herb may be used on occasion. Guidance is given about which part of the plant to use (e.g. weight of dried leaves or number of roots) and how to extract the active substances. For example, teas and decoctions are made by steeping the herbs in boiled water and then taking in cup or half-cup doses. Tinctures involve steeping the plants in alcohol for several weeks. The dose may be drops or teaspoons of the strained fluid.

Herbal recipes can be found in herbal self-help manuals and mixtures for brewing and ready-made tinctures are available through mail order. However, herbs must be used with care. They can have powerful effects that require specialist knowledge. For example, women with breast cancer should avoid certain herbs. Also, herbs are not without side-effects and may be of variable quality. Some countries have a tradition of using herbal medicine and have licensed products (Germany, France and now Australia), but herbs are unlicensed in the UK. This means that suppliers have no legal liability for their effects. These are some of the reasons why women may prefer to seek qualified advice from a herbalist and are advised to let their GP know what they plan to use.

Figure 12.2 Making sense of supplements

There are many menopause supplements available in chemists, health-food shops and from mail-order suppliers listed in the back of magazines. Here is a brief guide to some of the most common ingredients found in menopause formulas or sold separately.

- **Dong quai (*Angelica sinesis*).** Also known as tang kuei. Dong quai root is used widely in Chinese herbal medicine. It contains the plant oestrogen coumarin, but herbalists see dong quai as having a blood-harmonizing role. The herb can be strong, so use with care, especially when brewed. Side-effects include nausea and a hyperactive feeling.[10]
- **Wild yam (*Dioscorea*).** Wild yam has received a lot of attention in the media, often because it has been confused with natural progesterone. Wild yam contains the substance diosgenin which may be described on the tub as a 'chemical precursor' of hormones found in the body. This is potentially misleading (see Figure 11.1). Wild yam is sold as a supplement or a skin cream, but herbalists prefer brewing the roots for use as a

hormonal balancer. The roots have been found to be mildly oestrogenic.[11]

- **Black cohosh (*Cimicifuga racemosa*).** Black cohosh has some oestrogenic activity.[12] However, Remifemin, a black cohosh supplement, has been investigated as a remedy for hot flushes with conflicting results. Herbalists use the root in menopause brews for its stress-relieving properties. Black cohosh can cause unexpected bleeding and is not recommended for women with fibroids, which may be exacerbated.

- **Siberian ginseng (*Eleutherococcus senticosus*).** Used in one of the Chinese menopause formulas to reduce hot flushes, ginseng is also reported to produce changes in the vaginal lining and improve blood lipoprotein levels. May cause an unnerved feeling.

- **Chaste tree (*Vitex agnus-castus*).** This was reputedly used by nuns – hence its name. The berries have been shown to act on the pituitary gland. It is advised for a variety of menstrual problems as well as hot flushes. It is a strong but slow-acting herb to be used with care.

- **St John's Wort (*Hypericum perforatum*).** Sometimes described as the 'sunshine' herb, recent research has found this to be more effective than placebo for mild to moderate depression.[13] Women may or may not want such a substance in a menopause formulation, so check the ingredients. It is also sold widely as a separate supplement. This herb can take up to a month to help and may produce skin reactions.

- **Vitamin D.** Only women who are housebound are likely to lack Vitamin D, because sunlight on the skin enables the body to synthesize enough to help maintain bone. An estimated 15 minutes a day is all that is required. Dietary sources include mackerel, fish oils, eggs and milk. Vitamin D is often added to margarines. The recommended daily allowance is 5 mcg.

- **Vitamin E.** Appears to be better than placebo at reducing hot flushes in some women and levels of 100 iu/day may reduce the risk of heart disease. A little Vitamin E oil rubbed into the vagina regularly is often recommended for vaginal dryness, although it may take several weeks to have an effect. Vitamin E can be found in legumes, wholegrain cereal and rice, almonds, peanuts, unrefined vegetable oils and egg yolks. Taking Vitamin E supplements appears to be safe for women with breast cancer.[14]

- **Zinc.** Important mineral that enables the work of the immune system, prostaglandins and many enzymes, including those involved in Vitamin D and calcium pathways in bone. Often women are deficient because the body cannot store zinc and it is lowered by taking hormones. Oysters are the most frequently quoted, if not entirely practical, source of zinc. It is found in seafood, eggs, green vegetables and pumpkin seeds too. 15 mg/day is the recommended daily allowance.
- **Magnesium.** Necessary for calcium and bone metabolism. Magnesium deficiency is associated with bone loss (and other problems such as menstrual migraine). Magnesium can be taken as supplements (300 mg/day). Dietary sources include nuts, seafood, grapefruit, figs, dark vegetables, soy and other legumes and cereals.

Calcium

Current guidance is that women in the menopause should have 1500 mg/day of calcium unless they are on HRT, when 1000 mg/day is said to be sufficient. Women are advised to get this from their diet rather than using supplements. Calcium can be gained from soy foods, dairy products, sardines, leafy dark green vegetables, nuts and sesame seeds. For example, 2 oz (56 g) tofu contains 700 g; ⅓ pint of milk or 2 oz (56 g) sardines provides about 250 mg. Spinach and broccoli are other useful choices. Skimming milk does not reduce its calcium, so women can use skimmed and low-fat dairy products – although watch for hidden sugar in fruit yoghurts. Tahini, a sesame seed purée used in vegetarian cooking, is very high in calcium. Sesame seeds can be added to stir-fries or toasted and sprinkled over a green salad.

Calcium supplements come as ordinary, chewable or soluble tablets and 'fruit' powders. The latter may avoid side-effects such as constipation or diarrhoea. Most contain calcium carbonate (chalk), although some specialists recommend calcium citrate, which is absorbed more readily. One's calcium intake should not add up to more than 2 g/day.

Evening Primrose Oil (EPO)

Evening primrose oil is a good source of gamma-linolenic acid (GLA) and linoleic acid (LA). These names may ring a bell because they are both omega-6 essential fatty acids. They can also be found in other commercial products such as starflower (borage) oil and blackcurrant seed oil.

There are few studies of the effects of evening primrose oil on menopausal symptoms. One small investigation compared the experiences of women taking 2×1000 mg/day with those taking a placebo over six months. It found that evening primrose oil was better than placebo at reducing night sweats, but not day-time flushes.[15]

Nevertheless, evening primrose oil may benefit women who suffer from breast tenderness (mastalgia) as a side-effect of HRT. Often this side-effect occurs in the first few months and then wears off, so EPO can help women over this stage if they wish or need to continue using hormones. However, women will have to take a high dose of evening primrose oil for it to be effective. For instance, one study compared 3 g/day EPO (240 mg GLA) with two drugs commonly used for mastalgia (unrelated to HRT) and reported favourable results and fewer side-effects.[16] Diuretics and Vitamin B6 are no more effective than placebo for this problem.

Evening primrose oil is available on prescription, although this may not be a financial advantage. Anyone who wants to try it for themselves will find it in supermarkets, chemists or health-food shops. Look out for a 'high-strength' brand of evening primrose oil alone (e.g. 1000 mg capsule), because those for premenstrual tension usually have smaller doses and it can be annoying to discover that one has to take six or even 12 capsules a day to reach the suggested 3 grams! Also, PMT formulations may include other ingredients that should not be taken in a multiple dose. Some tubs give the dose in milligrams (mg) of evening primrose oil; others also list the dose of GLA, the active ingredient. Alternatively, there is a new liquid form that can be taken in a teaspoon.

Figure 12.3 Trouble-shooting guide to hot flushes

- Jot down when hot flushes occur and try to spot whether anything is acting as a trigger. Stress is often the culprit, but it may be alcohol, caffeine, spicy foods, garlic or other factors, like being in a confined space.
- Try a simple routine of slow deep breathing; pace it with counting or a favourite saying. It may help to practise this so that it is easier to call on it when necessary. Deep breathing has been found to be more effective than muscle relaxation techniques.[17]
- Research suggests that rooms at 19°C reduce the frequency and intensity of flushes compared to rooms at 31°C.[18] In other words, opt for cooler rooms, where possible.
- Choose clothes, night-clothes and bed-clothes in natural fibres, where possible.
- Plan to wear layers so that they can be shed easily and without extra stress and embarrassment.
- Make up the following blend of aromatherapy oils: 10 drops of clary sage, 11 drops of geranium, 7 drops of lemon and 2 drops of sage.[19] Use 5 drops of the blend in a bath or add the formula to 30 ml vegetable oil for massage.
- Steep 1 teaspoon of garden sage in a cup of boiled water; strain and sip.
- Choose to come off HRT with medical advice slowly, during winter and when nothing special is planned.

Aromatherapy

Aromatherapy uses essential oils derived from plants, some of which are said to be oestrogenic. However, aromatherapy oils have other properties that can help with menopausal symptoms, promote relaxation and enable sleep.

Traditionally essential oils are produced by extracting the 'essence' of a plant with boiling water and collecting the volatile substances, which rise with steam. Drops of the concentrated oil can then be added to a carrier oil for body massage or simply dispersed in a bath. They can also be inhaled when placed in a small diffuser sold for the purpose. Alternatively a few drops can be put in a bowl of hot water or placed on a tissue. Essential oils should not be taken by mouth and, with one or two exceptions, they should not be used neat on the skin (some oils should not be used in pregnancy).

The essential oils that are said to be oestrogenic are fennel, niaouli, aniseed, sage and clary sage. In addition, lemon is reputed to affect the hypothalamus and pituitary; peppermint the ovaries; peppermint, clove bud and thyme the uterus. The substances behind the oestrogenic qualities of certain oils are not well understood. However, researchers have noted that the compounds sclareol in clary-sage oil and viridiflorol in niaouli have similar structures to oestrogen and can influence the hormonal system.[20] Animal experiments have shown that fennel-seed extract can have slight oestrogenic effects.

Although the small bottles of essential oils have become a familiar sight in chemists, health-food and gift shops, many of these oils have been produced commercially for the food and perfume industries for many years. However, this production can mean that the oils are treated in ways that reduce the oils' merits in aromatherapy. According to one distributor, many cheap essential oils have had ingredients extracted or alcohol added and it is particularly difficult to get niaouli, one of the oestrogenic oils, in an unadulterated form.[21]

It is not easy to spot poor-quality oils, although there are certain things that might arouse one's suspicion. For example, expect a supplier's range to vary in price depending on the availability of the plant source and ease of production.[22] Also, pure essential oils do not leave an oily patch on blotting paper when they evaporate.

Homoeopathic Remedies

Homoeopathy is based on several important principles. Firstly, instead of being chosen for their ability to suppress symptoms, homoeopathic remedies are chosen because they *cause* the same symptoms in a healthy person. This is the homoeopathic 'law of similars'. The aim is to promote the body's own healing and, in that sense, the remedies are meant to start the ball rolling rather than be used long-term. However, several remedies might be tried as part of an exploratory process of matching the symptoms more closely. This process explains why homoeopaths will ask detailed questions about one's experience of the problem. As they point out, people experience the same disturbance in different ways and these variations are important if one is trying to match a remedy to the whole person.

The remedies are prepared from plants or minerals according to the homoeopathic principle of repeated dilution and 'succussion' (vigorous shaking). This method was devised by Samuel Hahnemann, an eighteenth-century physician, who was so alarmed by the side-effects of treatments used in medicine at the time that he was concerned to find the lowest effective doses. This led him to the surprising conclusion that even extreme dilutions produce results as long as they are shaken. A study in the scientific journal *Nature* suggested that vigorous shaking might 'imprint' the active substance on to the water molecules, enabling them to act long after the substance itself was diluted out, but its research methods have been hotly disputed.[23]

Homoeopathic remedies can be found in chemists and health-food shops with some advice on how to match them. Mail-order suppliers offer a wider choice. Potency is given as 30c or 6c, which refers to dilution on a 'c' or 100 scale. There is also a 'd' or 10 scale. The 100 scale is the more potent of the two because it is more diluted; 30c is more potent than 6c for the same reason. Beginners are advised to start with 6c.[24] The little tablets are meant to be sucked rather than swallowed and one is advised to avoid handling or contaminating them in any way. This includes avoiding interference from food, drink, sweets, cigarettes or toothpaste either before or after absorbing a remedy.

The remedies recommended for the menopause include sepia, belladonna, pulsatilla, lachesis, valeriana and sulphur. Detailed guidance on matching symptoms is available in various self-help guides or one can consult a homoeopath for an experienced assessment and advice on remedies that act more deeply than those available over the counter.

Finding an Alternative Practitioner

A practitioner can be found by writing to the relevant national organization for a list of practitioners (see More Help). Some organizations have registered members and a code of practice. However, alternative practitioners do not have to be registered to practise in the UK, unlike in the USA and elsewhere in Europe. This means that although they have a legal duty of care, there may be little chance of proving negligence if problems arise. Women are advised to check that practitioners carry indemnity insurance.

Now some GPs will refer patients for therapies such as osteopathy or homoeopathy. However, until recently GPs were not allowed to delegate patient care to medically unqualified staff and many are still reluctant to do so. This is partly because they remain clinically responsible when they make a referral. Most alternative therapies are not available on the NHS.

NOTES

2 BODY CHEMISTRY

1 Martin, E. (1987), *The Woman in the Body*, Open University Press
2 Chamberlain, G. V. P. (ed.) (1995), *Gynaecology by Ten Teachers*, Edward Arnold

3 NATURAL MENOPAUSE

1 Ginsburg, J. (1991), 'What determines the age at menopause?', *British Medical Journal*, 302, 1288–9 *and* Speroff, L. (1995), 'Premature ovarian failure', *Advances in Endocrinology and Metabolism*, 6, 233–58
2 Anasti, J. N. (1998), 'Premature ovarian failure: an update', *Fertility and Sterility*, 70 (1), 1–15
3 Ginsburg, 'What determines the age at menopause?'
4 Rees, M. C. P. (1997), 'Menstrual problems' in McPherson, A. and Waller, D. (eds), *Women's Health*, Oxford University Press
5 Coope, J. (1997), 'The menopause' in McPherson and Waller, *Women's Health*
6 Prelevic, G. M. and Jacobs, H. S. (1997), 'Menopause and post-menopause', *Baillière's Clinical Endocrinology and Metabolism*, 11 (2), 311–40
7 Coope, 'The menopause' in McPherson and Waller, *Women's Health*
8 Speroff, 'Premature ovarian failure'
9 Reviewed in Richardson, S. J. (1993), 'The biological basis of the menopause', *Baillière's Clinical Endocrinology and Metabolism*, 7 (1), 1–16
10 Melbourne Mid-Life Project, cited in Burger, H. G. (1996), 'The menopausal transition', *Baillière's Clinical Obstetrics and Gynaecology*, 10 (3), 347–59
11 Reviewed in Burger, 'The menopausal transition'

12 Kuh, D. L. et al. (1997), 'Women's health in mid-life: the influence of the menopause, social factors and health in earlier life', *British Journal of Obstetrics and Gynaecology*, 104, 923–33

13 Avis, N. E. et al. (1993), 'The evolution of menopausal symptoms', *Baillière's Clinical Endocrinology and Metabolism*, 7 (1), 17–32

14 Coope, 'The menopause' in McPherson and Waller, *Women's Health*

15 Liao, K. et al. (1994), 'Beliefs about the menopause of general practitioners and mid-aged women', *Family Practice*, 11 (4), 408–12

16 Whitehead, M. and Godfree, V. (1992), *HRT: Your Questions Answered*, Churchill Livingstone

17 Coope, 'The menopause' in McPherson and Waller, *Women's Health*

18 Prelevic and Jacobs, 'Menopause and post-menopause'

19 Freedman, R. R. (1998), 'Biochemical, metabolic and vascular mechanisms in menopausal hot flashes', *Fertility and Sterility*, 70 (2), 332–7

20 Shaw, C. (1997), 'The perimenopausal hot flash: epidemiology, physiology and treatment', *Nurse Practitioner*, 22 (3), 55–66

21 Whitehead and Godfree, *HRT: Your Questions Answered*

22 Ibid.

23 Hunter, M. S. (1993), 'Predictors of menopausal symptoms – psychosocial aspects', *Baillière's Clinical Endocrinology and Metabolism*, 7 (1), 33–46

24 Coope, 'The menopause' in McPherson and Waller, *Women's Health*

25 Pearce, M.-J. and Hawton, K. (1996), 'Psychological and sexual aspects of the menopause and HRT', *Baillière's Clinical Obstetrics and Gynaecology*, 10 (3), 385–99

26 Reviewed in Pearce and Hawton, 'Psychological and sexual aspects of the menopause and HRT'

27 Tang, M.-X. et al. (1996), 'Effect of oestrogen during menopause on risk and age at onset of Alzheimer's disease', *Lancet*, 348, 429–32

28 Hunter, M. S. (1996), 'Depression and the menopause', *British Medical Journal*, 313, 1217–18

29 Reviewed in Pearce and Hawton, 'Psychological and sexual aspects of the menopause and HRT'

30 Cawood, E. H. H. and Bancroft, J. (1996), 'Steroid hormones, the menopause, sexuality and well-being of women', *Psychological Medicine*, 26, 925–36

31 A'Court, C. et al. (1997), 'Complementary medicine and women's health' in McPherson and Waller, *Women's Health*

32 Whitehead and Godfree, *HRT: Your Questions Answered*

4 HORMONE REPLACEMENT THERAPY

1 Cited in Panay, N. and Studd, J. (1997), 'HRT after hysterectomy' in Studd, J. and Edwards, L. (eds), *Hysterectomy and HRT*, RCOG Press

2 Schaffer, J. and Fantl, J. A. (1996), 'Urogenital effects of the menopause', *Baillière's Clinical Obstetrics and Gynaecology*, 10 (3), 401–17

3 Coope, J. (1997), 'The menopause' in McPherson, A. and Waller, D. (eds), *Women's Health*, Oxford University Press

4 Schneider, H. P. G. (1996), 'The impact of different HRT regimens on compliance', *International Journal of Fertility*, 41 (1), 29–39

5 Whitehead, M. and Godfree, V. (1992), *HRT: Your Questions Answered*, Churchill Livingstone

6 Ibid.

7 Ibid.

8 Gladwell, M. (1997), 'The estrogen question', *New Yorker*, June 9

9 Whitehead and Godfree, *HRT: Your Questions Answered*

10 Schneider, 'The impact of different HRT regimens on compliance'

11 Bush, T. L. (1996), 'Evidence for primary and secondary prevention of coronary artery disease in women taking oestrogen replacement therapy', *European Heart Journal*, 17, Supp. D, 9–14

12 Coope, 'The menopause' in McPherson and Waller, *Women's Health*

13 Whitehead and Godfree, *HRT: Your Questions Answered*

14 Hartmann, B. W. and Huber, J. C. (1997), 'The mythology of hormone replacement therapy', *British Journal of Obstetrics and Gynaecology*, 104, 163–8

15 *British National Formulary*, 35 (March 1998)

16 Coope, 'The menopause' in McPherson and Waller, *Women's Health*

17 Whitehead, M. (1996), 'Treatments for menopausal and post-menopausal problems: present and future', *Baillière's Clinical Obstetrics and Gynaecology*, 10 (3), 515–30

18 Rako, S. (1996), *The Hormone of Desire: The Truth about Menopause, Sexuality and Testosterone*, Harmony Books

19 Hoberman, J. M. and Yesalis, C. E. (1995), 'The history of synthetic testosterone', *Scientific American*, February, 60–65

20 Davis, S. R. and Burger, H. G. (1996), 'Androgens and the postmenopausal woman', *Journal of Clinical Endocrinology and Metabolism*, 81 (8), 2759–63

21 Casson, P. R. and Casson, S. A. (1996), 'Androgen replacement therapy in women: myths and realities', *International Journal of Fertility*, 41 (4), 412–22

22 Davis and Burger, 'Androgens and the postmenopausal woman'

23 Sherwin, B. B. (1997), 'The use of androgens in the postmenopause: evidence from clinical studies' in Wren, B. G. (ed.), *Progress in the Management of the Menopause*, Parthenon

24 Cited in Hoberman and Yesalis, 'The history of synthetic testosterone'

25 Compston, J. E. (1997), 'Designer oestrogens: fact or fantasy?', *Lancet*, 350, 676–7

5 HEART DISEASE, OSTEOPOROSIS AND BREAST CANCER

1 McConway, K. (ed.) (1994), *Studying Health and Disease*, Open University Press

2 Barrett-Connor, E. (1998), 'Hormone replacement therapy', *British Medical Journal*, 317, 457–61

3 McPherson, K. (1995), 'Breast cancer and hormonal supplements in postmenopausal women', *British Medical Journal*, 311, 699–700

4 Wren, B. G. (1996), 'The breast and the menopause', *Baillière's Clinical Obstetrics and Gynaecology*, 10 (3), 433–47

5 Collaborative Group on Hormonal Factors in Breast Cancer (1997), 'Breast cancer and hormone replacement therapy', *Lancet*, 350, 1047–59

6 Horton, R. (1997), 'ICRF: from mayhem to meltdown', *Lancet*, 350, 1043–4

7 Sullivan, J. M. and Fowlkes, L. P. (1996), 'The clinical aspects of estrogen

and the cardiovascular system', *Obstetrics and Gynecology*, 87 (2), Supp. 36S–43S

8 Bush, T. (1996), 'Evidence for primary and secondary prevention of coronary artery disease in women taking oestrogen replacement therapy', *European Heart Journal*, 17, Supp. D, 9–14

9 Schenck-Gustafsson, K. (1996), 'Risk factors for cardiovascular disease in women: assessment and management', *European Heart Journal*, 17, Supp. D, 2–8

10 Vyas, S. and Gangar, K. (1995), 'Postmenopausal oestrogens and arteries', *British Journal of Obstetrics and Gynaecology*, 102, 942–6

11 Tunstall-Pedoe, H. (1998), 'Myth and paradox of coronary risk and the menopause', *Lancet*, 351, 1425–7

12 Wild, R. A. (1996), 'Estrogen: effects on the cardiovascular tree', *Obstetrics and Gynecology*, 87 (2), Supp. 27S–35S

13 Prelevic, G. M. and Jacobs, H. S. (1997), 'Menopause and post-menopause', *Baillière's Clinical Endocrinology and Metabolism*, 11 (2), 311–40

14 Lobo, R. A. and Speroff, L. (1994), 'International consensus conference on post-menopausal hormone therapy and the cardiovascular system', *Fertility and Sterility*, 62 (6), Supp. 2, 176S–180S

15 Grodstein, F. et al. (1997), 'Postmenopausal hormone therapy and mortality', *New England Journal of Medicine*, 336 (25), 1769–822

16 Newnham, H. H. and Silberberg, J. (1997), 'Women's hearts are hard to break', *Lancet*, 349, sI3–sI6

17 McPherson, A. and Waller, D. (1997), 'Women's health and its controversies – an overview' in McPherson, A. and Waller, D. (eds), *Women's Health*, Oxford University Press

18 Hulley, S. et al. (1998), 'Randomized trial of estrogen plus progestin for secondary prevention of coronary heart disease in postmenopausal women', *Journal of the American Medical Association*, 280 (7), 605–13

19 Eastell, R. (1998), 'Treatment of postmenopausal osteoporosis', *New England Journal of Medicine*, 338 (11), 737–46

20 Kanis, J. A. (1996), 'The menopause and the skeleton: key issues', *Baillière's Clinical Obstetrics and Gynaecology*, 10 (3), 469–82

21 Li. Mosekilde and Thomsen, J. S. (1997), 'Bone structure and function in

relation to ageing and the menopause' in Wren, B. G. (ed.), *Progress in the Management of the Menopause*, Parthenon

22 Rizzoli, R. and Bonjour, J. (1997), 'Hormones and bones', *Lancet*, 349, s120–s123

23 Lindsay, R. (1996), 'Menopause and osteoporosis', *Obstetrics and Gynecology*, 87 (2), Supp., 16S–19S

24 Steering Group (1992), 'Screening for osteoporosis to prevent fractures', *Effective Health Care*, 1, 1–10

25 Eriksen, E. F. (1997), 'Clinical aspects of estrogens and osteoporosis' in Wren, *Progress in the Management of the Menopause*

26 Department of Health (1998), *Strategy to Prevent and Tackle Osteoporosis: Information for NHS Professionals and Health Organisations*

27 Stern, P. H. et al. (1997), 'Estrogens and bone cells' in Wren, *Progress in the Management of the Menopause*

28 Eriksen, 'Clinical aspects of estrogens and osteoporosis' in Wren, *Progress in the Management of the Menopause*

29 Barrett-Connor, 'Hormone replacement therapy'

30 Khaw, K. (1998), 'Hormone replacement therapy again', *British Medical Journal*, 316, 1842–3

31 Rizzoli and Bonjour, 'Hormones and bones'

32 Barrett-Connor, 'Hormone replacement therapy'

33 Newnham and Silberberg, 'Women's hearts are hard to break'

34 Rizzoli and Bonjour, 'Hormones and bones'

35 Coope, J. (1997), 'The menopause' in McPherson and Waller, *Women's Health*

36 McPherson and Waller, 'Women's health and its controversies – an overview' in McPherson and Waller, *Women's Health*

37 Wren, 'The breast and the menopause'

38 Collaborative Group on Hormonal Factors in Breast Cancer. 'Breast cancer and hormone replacement therapy'

39 Cohen, M. E. L. (1997), 'Effect of HRT on cancer detection by mammography', *Lancet*, 349, 1624

40 Barrett-Connor, 'Hormone replacement therapy'

41 Austoker, J. et al. (1997), 'Breast problems' in McPherson and Waller, *Women's Health*

6 INTERRUPTED SEXUAL DEVELOPMENT

1 Sadler, T. W. (1995), *Langman's Medical Embryology*, 7th edition, Williams & Wilkins

2 Zajac, J. D. and Warne, G. L. (1995), 'Disorders of sexual development', *Baillière's Clinical Endocrinology and Metabolism*, 9 (3), 555–80

3 Saenger, P. (1996), 'Turner's syndrome', *New England Journal of Medicine*, 335 (23), 1749–54 *and* Ogata, T. et al. (1995), 'Turner syndrome and female sex chromosome aberrations', *Human Genetics*, 95, 607–29 quoting Loughlin, S. A. R. et al. review 1991

4 Davis, S. R. (1996), 'Premature ovarian failure', *Maturitas*, 23, 1–8

5 Saenger, 'Turner's syndrome'

6 Kim, H. H. and Laufer, M. R. (1994), 'Developmental abnormalities of the female reproductive tract', *Current Opinion in Obstetrics and Gynecology*, 6, 518–25

7 Lanson, L. (1983), *From Woman to Woman*, Penguin

8 Kim and Laufer, 'Developmental abnormalities of the female reproductive tract'

9 Informal reports from Internet MRKH online support group (1999) and case report in Cramer, D. W. et al. (1987), *Fertility and Sterility*, 'Müllerian aplasia', 47 (6), 930–34

10 Fox, S. I. (1996), *Human Physiology*, 5th edition, W. C. Brown

11 Kim and Laufer, 'Developmental abnormalities of the female reproductive tract'

12 ALIAS 1 (2), summer 1995, AIS Support Group newsletter

13 ALIAS 1 (11), spring 1998, AIS Support Group newsletter

14 Discussion at UK Turner Society Open Day, 21 February 1998

15 Kagan-Krieger, S. (1998), *The Struggle to Understand Oneself as a Woman: Stress, Coping and the Psychological Development of Women with Turner Syndrome*, unpublished doctoral thesis, OISE/University of Toronto

16 Vockrodt, L. et al. (1994), 'A reproductive option for women with Turner's syndrome', *Journal of Pediatric Nursing*, 9 (5), 321–5

17 For detailed recommendations, see Kagan-Krieger, *The Struggle to Understand Oneself as a Woman*

18 Masters, K. W. (1996), 'Treatment of Turner's syndrome – a concern', *Lancet*, 348, 681–2 *and* Conway, G. S., Davies, M. and Merry, A. (1996), 'Treatment of Turner's syndrome', *Lancet*, 348, 1590–91

19 Masters, 'Treatment of Turner's syndrome – a concern' *and* Conway, Davies and Merry, 'Treatment of Turner's syndrome – a concern'

20 Cited in Kagan-Krieger, *The Struggle to Understand Oneself as a Woman*

21 Saenger, 'Turner syndrome'

22 Kagan-Krieger, *The Struggle to Understand Oneself as a Woman*

23 Unpublished PhD thesis in progress, Kathy Mill, University of Western Sydney

24 Papers cited in Davies, M. C. et al. (1995), 'Osteoporosis in Turner's syndrome and other forms of primary amenorrhoea', *Clinical Endocrinology*, 43, 741–6

25 Cited in Zajac and Warne, 'Disorders of sexual development'

26 Discussion in ALIAS 1 (11), spring 1998 and back issues of AIS Support Group newsletter

27 Patterson, M. N. et al. (1994), 'Androgen insensitivity syndrome', *Baillière's Clinical Endocrinology and Metabolism*, 8 (2), 379–404

28 Soule, S. G. et al. (1995), 'Osteopenia as a feature of the androgen insensitivity syndrome', *Clinical Endocrinology*, 43, 671–5 and discussion in ALIAS 1 (6), winter 1996

7 PREMATURE MENOPAUSE

1 Coulam, C. B., Adamson, S. C. and Annegers, J. F. (1986), 'Incidence of premature ovarian failure', *Obstetrics and Gynecology*, 67 (4), 604–6

2 Cited in Hoek, A. et al. (1997), 'Premature ovarian failure and ovarian autoimmunity', *Endocrine Reviews*, 18 (1), 107–34

3 Reviewed in Hoek, 'Premature ovarian failure and ovarian autoimmunity'

4 Cited in Davis, S. R. (1996), 'Premature ovarian failure', *Maturitas*, 23, 1–8

5 Cited in Barlow, D. H. (1996), 'Premature ovarian failure', *Baillière's Clinical Obstetrics and Gynaecology*, 10 (3), 361–84

6 Davis, 'Premature ovarian failure'

7 Hoek et al. (1997), 'Premature ovarian failure and ovarian autoimmunity'

8 Barlow, 'Premature ovarian failure'

9 Davis, 'Premature ovarian failure'

10 Warren, M. (1996), 'Evaluation of secondary amenorrhea', *Journal of Clinical Endocrinology and Metabolism*, 81 (2), 437–42

11 Conway, G. S. et al. (1996), 'Characterization of idiopathic premature ovarian failure', *Fertility and Sterility*, 65 (2), 337–41

12 Barlow, 'Premature ovarian failure'

13 Conway, 'Characterization of idiopathic premature ovarian failure'

14 Warren, 'Evaluation of secondary amenorrhea'

15 Schwartz, C. et al. (1994), 'Obstetric and gynaecological complications in fragile X carriers', *American Journal of Human Genetics*, 51, 400–402 *and* Conway, G. S. et al. (1995), 'Fragile X premutations in familial premature ovarian failure, *Lancet*, 346, 309–10

16 Reviews cited in Barlow, 'Premature ovarian failure'

17 Conway et al., 'Characterization of idiopathic premature ovarian failure'

18 Ibid.

19 Wheatcroft, N. J. et al. (1997), 'Identification of ovarian antibodies by immunofluorescence, enzyme-linked immunosorbent assay or immunoblotting in premature ovarian failure', *Human Reproduction*, December 12 (12), 2617–22

20 Adapted from Lockwood, G. M. (1997), 'Infertility and early pregnancy loss' in McPherson, A. and Waller, D. (eds), *Women's Health*, Oxford University Press

21 Pados, G. et al. (1992), cited in Barlow, 'Premature ovarian failure'

22 Davis, 'Premature ovarian failure'

8 SURGICAL AND MEDICAL MENOPAUSE

1 Austoker, J. et al. (1997), 'Breast problems' in McPherson, A. and Waller, D. (eds), *Women's Health*, Oxford University Press

2 Herod, J. J. O. et al. (1997), 'Hysterectomy and HRT' in Studd, J. W. W. and Edwards, L. (eds), *Hysterectomy and HRT*, RCOG Press

3 Vessey, M. P. et al. (1992), 'The epidemiology of hysterectomy: findings

in a large cohort study', *British Journal of Obstetrics and Gynaecology*, 99, 402–7

4 Pokras, R. and Hufnagel, V. (1988), 'Hysterectomy in the United States 1965–84', *American Journal of Public Health*, 78, 852–64

5 Li, T. C. and Saravelos, H. (1994), 'Oophorectomy at the same time as hysterectomy', *British Journal of Obstetrics and Gynaecology*, November, 101, 934–6

6 Whitehead, M. and Godfree, V. (1992), *HRT: Your Questions Answered*, Churchill Livingstone

7 Norman, S. G. and Studd, J. W. W. (1994), 'A survey of views on hormone replacement therapy', *British Journal of Obstetrics and Gynaecology*, October, 101, 879–87

8 e.g. Hufnagel, V. G. with Golant, S. K. (1989), *No More Hysterectomies*, Plume

9 Rees, M. C. P. (1997), 'Menstrual problems' in McPherson and Waller, *Women's Health*

10 Vessey et al., 'The epidemiology of hysterectomy: findings in a large cohort study'

11 Norman and Studd, 'A survey of views on hormone replacement therapy'

12 Siddle, N., Sarrell, P. and Whitehead, M. (1987), 'The effect of hysterectomy on the age of ovarian failure', *Fertility and Sterility*, 47 (1), 94–100

13 Brahams, D. (1997), 'UK gynaecologist found guilty of serious professional misconduct', *Lancet*, 350, 1014 *and* Dyer, C. (1998), 'Gynaecologist showed "lack of care and judgement"', *British Medical Journal*, 317, 965

14 Cited in Panay, N. and Studd, J. (1997), 'HRT after hysterectomy' in Studd, J. and Edwards, L. (eds), *Hysterectomy and HRT*, RCOG Press

15 Peterson, C. M. (1995), 'The rational use of androgens in hormone replacement therapy', *Clinical Obstetrics and Gynecology*, 38 (4), 915–20

16 RCOG (1994), *Endometriosis*, Gynaecology Information Pamphlet, RCOG Press

17 Hartmann, B. W. and Huber, J. C. (1997), 'The mythology of hormone replacement therapy', *British Journal of Obstetrics and Gynaecology*, 104, 163–8

18 Eeles, R. A. et al. (1991), 'HRT and survival after surgery for ovarian cancer', *British Medical Journal*, 302, 259–62

19 Sherwin, B. B. et al. cited in Pearce, M.-J. and Hawton, K. (1996), 'Psychological and sexual aspects of the menopause and HRT', *Baillière's Clinical Obstetrics and Gynaecology*, 10 (3), 385–99

20 Casson, P. R. and Casson, S. A. (1996), 'Androgen replacement therapy in women: myths and realities', *International Journal of Fertility*, 41 (4), 412–22

21 Spector, T. D. (1989), 'Use of oestrogen replacement therapy in high-risk groups in the UK', *British Medical Journal*, 229, 1434–5

22 Edwards, L. (1997), 'The woman's perspective of hysterectomy' in Studd and Edwards, *Hysterectomy and HRT*

23 Norman and Studd, 'A survey of views on hormone replacement therapy'

24 Edwards, 'The woman's perspective of hysterectomy' in Studd and Edwards, *Hysterectomy and HRT*

25 Anasti, J. N. (1998), 'Premature ovarian failure: an update', *Fertility and Sterility*, 70 (1), 1–15

26 Cited in Warren, M. (1996), 'Evaluation of secondary amenorrhea', *Journal of Clinical Endocrinology and Metabolism*, 81 (2), 437–42

27 Anasti, 'Premature ovarian failure'

28 Cited in Barlow, D. H. (1996), 'Premature ovarian failure', *Baillière's Clinical Obstetrics and Gynaecology*, 10 (3), 361–84

29 Craighead, M. (1986), *The Mother's Songs*, Paulist Press

9 WHY DOCTORS CAN'T AGREE ABOUT HRT (AND WOMEN CAN'T EITHER)

1 Toozs-Hobson, P. and Cardozo, L. (1996), 'HRT for all? Universal prescription desirable', *British Medical Journal*, 313, 350–51

2 For example, speaker at National Osteoporosis Society meeting, Manchester, October 1996

3 Bewley, S. (1996), 'HRT for all? Arguments should be based on ratio of benefits to risks', *British Medical Journal*, 313, 1205–6 *and* Lock, M. (1998), 'Postmenopausal body', *Body and Society*, 4 (1), 35–61

4 Davey, B. and Halliday, T. (eds) (1994), *Human Biology and Health: An Evolutionary Approach*, Open University Press

5 Davey, B. (1995), *Birth to Old Age: Health in Transition*, Open University Press

6 Jacobs, H. (1996), 'Not for everybody', *British Medical Journal*, 313, 351–2

7 Bewley, S. and Bewley, T. H. (1992), 'Drug dependence with oestrogen replacement therapy', *Lancet*, 339, 290–91

8 Norman, S. G. and Studd, J. W. W. (1994), 'A survey of views on hormone replacement therapy', *British Journal of Obstetrics and Gynaecology*, 101, 879–87

9 Liao, K. et al. (1994), 'Beliefs about the menopause of general practitioners and mid-aged women', *Family Practice*, 11 (4), 408–12

10 Price, E. H. et al. (1997), 'Women need to be warned about the dangers of HRT', *British Medical Journal*, 314, 376–7, announcing DASH (Doctors Against Abuse of Steroid Hormones)

11 Ussher, J. M. (1989), *The Psychology of the Female Body*, Routledge

12 Orbach, S. (1978), *Fat is a Feminist Issue*, Arrow

13 Lock, M. (1991), 'Contested meanings of the menopause', *Lancet*, 337, 1270–72

14 Ussher, *The Psychology of the Female Body*

15 Liao et al., 'Beliefs about the menopause of general practitioners and mid-aged women'

16 Hunter, M. S. (1993), 'Predictors of menopausal symptoms: psychosocial aspects', *Baillière's Clinical Endocrinology and Metabolism*, 7 (1), 33–46

17 Coope, J. and Hunter, M. S. (1993), 'Impact of menopausal symptoms: effect on quality of life exaggerated', *British Medical Journal*, 307, 1420

18 Editorial (1975), 'Eternal youth', *Lancet*, June 7, 1282

19 J. B. McKinlay, director of the New England Research Institute, Watertown, Mass., quoted in Hoberman, J. M. and Yesalis, C. E. (1995), 'The history of synthetic testosterone', *Scientific American*, February, 60–65

20 Hunter, M. S. and Liao, K. L.-M. (1995), 'Determinants of treatment choice for menopausal hot flushes: hormonal versus psychological versus no treatment', *Journal of Psychosomatic Obstetrics and Gynecology*, 16, 101–8

21 Quoted by Stephen Jay Gould and cited by Greenhalgh, T. (1998),

'Research methods for primary care', *British Journal of General Practice*, June, 1356–7

22 Greenhalgh, T. (1998), 'Meta-analysis and beyond: applying secondary research methods to primary care', *British Journal of General Practice*, August, 1540–41

23 Jacobs, 'Not for everybody'

24 Coope, J. (1997), 'The menopause' in McPherson, A. and Waller, D. (eds), *Women's Health*, Oxford University Press

25 Horton, R. (1998), 'The *new* new public health of risk and radical engagement', *Lancet*, 352, 251–2

26 Lock, 'Postmenopausal body'

27 Lupton, D. (1993), 'Risk as moral danger: the social and political functions of risk discourse in public health', *International Journal of Health Services*, 23 (3), 425–35

28 Barlow, D. H. (1997), 'Who understands the menopause?', *British Journal of Obstetrics and Gynaecology*, 107, 879–80

10 USING HRT

1 Whitehead, M. and Godfree, V. (1992), *HRT: Your Questions Answered*, Churchill Livingstone

2 Cited in Jewelewicz, R. (1997), 'New developments in topical estrogen therapy', *Fertility and Sterility*, 67 (1), 1–12

3 Sturdee, D. (1997), 'Newer HRT regimes', *British Journal of Obstetrics and Gynaecology*, 104, 1109–15

4 Bewley, S. and Bewley, T. H. (1992), 'Drug dependence with oestrogen replacement therapy', *Lancet*, 339, 290–91

5 Panay, N. and Studd, J. (1997), 'HRT after hysterectomy' in Studd, J. W. W. and Edwards, L. (eds), *Hysterectomy and HRT*, RCOG Press

6 Garnett, T. et al. (1990), 'Hormone implants and tachyphylaxis', *British Journal of Obstetrics and Gynaecology*, 97, 917–21

7 Buckler, H. et al. (1995), 'An audit of oestradiol levels and implant frequency in women undergoing subcutaneous implant therapy', *Clinical Endocrinology*, 42, 445–50

8 Panay and Studd, 'HRT after hysterectomy' in Studd and Edwards, *Hysterectomy and HRT*

9 Coope, J. (1997), 'The menopause' in McPherson, A. and Waller, D. (eds), *Women's Health*, Oxford University Press

10 Sturdee, 'Newer HRT regimes'

11 *British National Formulary*, 35, March 1998

12 Coope, 'The menopause' in McPherson and Waller, *Women's Health*

13 RCOG (1994), *Endometriosis*, Gynaecology Information Pamphlets, RCOG Press

14 Sherwin, B. B. and Gelfand, M. M. cited in Casson, P. R. and Casson, S. A. (1996), 'Androgen replacement therapy in women: myths and realities', *International Journal of Fertility*, 41 (4), 412–22

15 Davis, S. R. and Burger, H. G. (1996), 'Androgens and the postmenopausal woman', *Journal of Clinical Endocrinology and Metabolism*, 81 (8), 2759–63

16 Casson and Casson, 'Androgen replacement therapy in women: myths and realities'

17 Sherwin, B. B. (1997), 'The use of androgens in the postmenopause: evidence from clinical studies' in Wren, B. G. (ed.), *Progress in the Management of the Menopause*, Parthenon

18 Rako, S. (1996), 'Testosterone deficiency and supplementation for women: what do we need to know?', *Menopause Management*, 5 (4), 10–15

19 Sherwin, 'The use of androgens in the postmenopause: evidence from clinical studies' in Wren, *Progress in the Management of the Menopause*

20 Casson and Casson, 'Androgen replacement therapy in women: myths and realities'

21 Buckler, H. M. and Robertson, W. R. (1997), 'Androgen production over the female life span' in Wren, *Progress in the Management of the Menopause*

22 Sturdee, 'Newer HRT regimes'

23 Schaffer, J. and Fantl, J. A. (1996), 'Urogenital effects of the menopause', *Baillière's Clinical Obstetrics and Gynaecology*, 10 (3), 401–17

24 Ibid.

25 Coope, 'The menopause' in McPherson and Waller, *Women's Health*

11 NATURAL PROGESTERONE

1 Lee, J. R. (1993), *Natural Progesterone: The Multiple Roles of a Remarkable Hormone*, Jon Carpenter Publishing

2 Ibid.

3 Lee, J. R. with Hopkins, V. (1996), *What Your Doctor May Not Tell You about Menopause: The Breakthrough Book on Natural Progesterone*, Warner Books

4 Lee, J. R. (1996), 'Osteoporosis reversal with transdermal progesterone' (letter), *Lancet*, 336, 1327

5 Natural Progesterone Information Service Factsheets

6 A'Court, C. et al. (1997), 'Complementary medicine and women's health' in McPherson, A. and Waller, D. (eds), *Women's Health*, Oxford University Press

7 Ibid.

8 Lee with Hopkins, *What Your Doctor May Not Tell You about Menopause*

9 Ibid.

10 Cooper, A. et al. (1998), 'Systemic absorption of progesterone from Pro-Gest cream in postmenopausal women', *Lancet*, 351, 1255–6

11 Smallbone, D. F. (1998), *The* Lancet *Report on Pro-Gest Cream Explained*, Natural Progesterone Information Service

12 Chamberlain, G. V. P. (ed.) (1995), *Gynaecology by Ten Teachers*, Edward Arnold

13 Glenville, M. (1997), *Natural Alternatives to HRT*, Kyle Cathie

14 McTaggart, L. (1997), *Guide to the Menopause*, What Doctors Don't Tell You Ltd

15 Lee with Hopkins, *What Your Doctor May Not Tell You about Menopause*

16 Glenville, *Natural Alternatives to HRT*

17 Wright, C. (1997), *How Safe is Natural Progesterone?*, Natural Progesterone Information Service, Factsheet 5

18 Glenville, *Natural Alternatives to HRT*

19 Natural Progesterone Information Service Factsheets

20 Royal College of Physicians debate on natural progesterone, National Osteoporosis Society newsletter, June 1998

21 'Miracles on demand' (1998), editorial in *New Scientist*, 22 August, 3

22 Lee with Hopkins, *What Your Doctor May Not Tell You about Menopause*

23 Mackenzie, D. (1998), 'A cure for quacks', *New Scientist*, 22 August, 18–19

12 OTHER ALTERNATIVES

1 Wilcox, G. (1997), 'The effect of soy on menopausal symptoms' in Wren, B. G. (ed.), *Progress in the Management of the Menopause*, Parthenon Publishing

2 Ibid.

3 A'Court, C. et al. (1997), 'Complementary medicine and women's health' in McPherson, A. and Waller, D. (eds), *Women's Health*, Oxford University Press

4 Lien, L. L. and Lien, E. J. (1996), 'Hormone therapy and phytoestrogens', *Journal of Clinical Pharmacy and Therapeutics*, 21, 101–11

5 Hughes, C. L. et al. (1997), 'Dietary soy phytoestrogens and the health of menopausal women' in Wren, *Progress in the Management of the Menopause*

6 Wilcox, 'The effect of soy on menopausal symptoms' in Wren, *Progress in the Management of the Menopause*

7 Ibid.

8 Ibid.

9 Lien and Lien, 'Hormone therapy and phytoestrogens'

10 Shaw, C. (1997), 'The perimenopausal hot flash: epidemiology, physiology and treatment', *Nurse Practitioner*, 22 (3), 55–66

11 Lien and Lien, 'Hormone therapy and phytoestrogens'

12 Ibid.

13 A'Court et al., 'Complementary medicine and women's health' in McPherson and Waller, *Women's Health*

14 Ibid.

15 Shaw, 'The perimenopausal hot flash: epidemiology, physiology and treatment'

16 A'Court et al., 'Complementary medicine and women's health' in McPherson and Waller, *Women's Health*

17 Cited in Coope, J. (1996), 'Hormonal and non-hormonal interventions for menopausal symptoms', *Maturitas*, 23, 159–68

18 Shaw, 'The perimenopausal hot flash: epidemiology, physiology and treatment'

19 Worwood, V. A. (1990), *The Fragrant Pharmacy*, Bantam Books

20 Price, S. and Price, L. (1995), *Aromatherapy for Health Professionals*, Churchill Livingstone

21 Ibid.

22 Worwood, *The Fragrant Pharmacy*

23 Davenas, E. et al. (1988), 'Human basophil degranulation triggered by very dilute antiserum against IgE', *Nature*, 333, 816–18 *and* Maddox, J. et al. (1988), ' "High dilution" experiments a delusion', *Nature*, 334, 287–91

24 MacEoin, B. (1995), *Homoeopathy and the Menopause*, Thorsons

MORE HELP

Further Reading

For a range of views:

The Menopause Industry, Sandra Coney, The Women's Press, 1995

The Menopause: Coping with the Change, Dr Jean Coope, Vermilion, 1997

Turning Point, C. Sue Furman, Oxford University Press, 1995

Natural Alternatives to HRT, Marilyn Glenville, Kyle Cathie, 1997

Sexual Chemistry, Dr Ellen Grant, Cedar, 1994 (available in libraries)

The Change: Women, Ageing and the Menopause, Germaine Greer, Penguin, 1993

What Your Doctors May Not Tell You about the Menopause: The Breakthrough Book on Natural Progesterone, Dr John Lee with Virginia Hopkins, Warner, 1996

The Hormone Dilemma, Dr Susan Love with Karen Lindsey, Thorsons, 1997

The Silent Passage, Gail Sheehy, HarperCollins, 1991

Useful Addresses

- The addresses given below are in the UK, unless otherwise specified.
- Organizations welcome a large stamp addressed envelope with inquiries.
- Some groups charge for leaflets or for a list of registered practitioners.

Details of relevant organizations can also be obtained by consulting local libraries for directories of charities and self-help groups. Increasingly libraries provide opportunities to use the Internet and Worldwide Web. UK helplines are also listed in places such as the Thomson Local Directory or call the freephone health information service on 0800 665544.

Amarant Trust
11–13 Charterhouse Buildings
London
EC1M 7AN
General helpline (recorded/call charges): 0891 660620
Premature Menopause Helpline (recorded/call charges): 0891 660632
Provides information and menopause counselling and treatment clinics.

Androgen Insensitivity Syndrome (AIS) Support Group
P.O. Box 269
Banbury
OX15 6YT
http://www.medhelp.org/www/ais (includes details of overseas branches)
Also provides support for those affected by Swyer's syndrome, 5-alpha-reductase deficiency, MRKH syndrome, Müllerian dysgenesis, Müllerian duct aplasia, vaginal atresia and related conditions.

British Acupuncture Council
Park House
206–208 Latimer Rd
London
W10 6RE
0181 964 0222

British Agencies for Adoption and Fostering (BAAF)
11 Southwark St
London
SE1 1RQ

CancerBACUP
3 Bath Place
Rivington St
London
EC2A 3JR
Information service: 0171 613 2121
Freephone: 0800 181199
http://www.cancerbacup.org.uk

Cancerlink
11–21 Northdown St
London
N1 9BN
Freephone helpline for young people: 0800 591028
Freephone information helpline: 0800 132905 (textphone available)
Freephone Asian information helpline: 0800 590415

CHILD (National Infertility Support Network)
Charter House
43 St Leonard's Rd
Bexhill-on-Sea
TN40 1JA
01424 732361
http://www.child.org.uk

Child Growth Foundation
2 Mayfield Avenue
London
W4 1PW
0181 994 7625 or 0181 995 0257
(Contact for parent/patient support groups for Growth Hormone Insufficiency, Turner Syndrome, IUGR/Russell Silver, Bone Dysplasia, Sotos and Premature Sexual Maturation.)

Congenital Adrenal Hyperplasia (CAH) Network
c/o Miss Melissa Cull
17 Newton Road
Lichfield
WS13 7EF
Adult/teen support: 01543 252961
Email: CAH.Network@mlcull.demon.co.uk

Continence Foundation
307 Hatton Square
16 Baldwins Gardens
London
EC1N 7RJ
0171 404 6875
Can provide information on pelvic floor exercises to prevent urinary incontinence.

Endometriosis Association (USA)
8585 N. 76th Place
Milwaukee
Wisconsin 53223
USA
http://www.endometriosisassn.org/
See also *National Endometriosis Society*

Foresight (Preconceptual Care)
28 The Paddock
Godalming
Surrey
GU7 1XD

Hodgkin's Disease and Lymphoma Association
P.O. Box 275
Haddenham
Aylesbury
HP17 8JJ
Helpline: 01844 291500
http://www.nhsconfed.net/hodgkins/

Human Fertilization and Embryological Authority (HFEA)
Paxton House
30 Artillery Lane
London
E1 7LS
0171 377 5077
Licenses and regulates IVF centres in the UK; also provides a guide to centres.
http://www.hfea.gov.uk/

Hysterectomy Association
Aynsley House
Chester Gardens
Church Gresley
Swadlincote
DE11 9PU
http://www.hysterectomy-association.org.uk/index.htm

Intersex Society of North America
P.O. Box 31791
San Francisco
California 94131
USA
http://www.isna.org/

ISSUE (National Fertility Association)
114 Lichfield Street
Walsall
WS1 1SZ
01922 722888
http://www.issue.co.uk

Leukaemia Care Society
14 Kingfisher Court
Venny Bridge
Pinhoe
Exeter
EX4 8JN
Helpline: 0345 673 2203

MacMillan Cancer Relief
15–19 Britten St
London
SW3 3TZ
Information line: 0845 601 6161

Mayer-Rokitansky-Kuster-Hauser (MRKH) Syndrome
Additional information (as well as an online support group) can be found
on the TASC (The American Surrogacy Center) website at:
http://www.surrogacy.com

Miscarriage Association
c/o Clayton Hospital
Northgate
Wakefield
WF1 3JS
01924 200799

National Endometriosis Society
Suite 50
Westminster Palace Gardens
1–7 Artillery Row
London
SW1P 1RL
Helpline (7–10 p.m. daily): 0171 222 2776

National Institute of Medical Herbalists
56 Longbrook St
Exeter
EX4 6AH
01392 426022

National Osteoporosis Foundation (USA)
1150 17th St
NW Suite 500
Washington DC 20036-4603
USA

National Osteoporosis Society
P.O. Box 10
Radstock
Bath
BA3 3YB
Helpline: 01761 472721

Natural Progesterone Information Service
P.O. Box 24
Buxton
SK17 9FB

Ovacome (Ovarian Cancer Support Network)
St Bartholomew's Hospital
West Smithfield
London
EC1A 7BE
07071 781861
http://dspace.dial.pipex.com/ovacome

Parent-to-Parent Information on Adoption Services (PPIAS)
Lower Boddington
Daventry
Northampton
NN11 6 YB
0327 60295

Patients' Association
P.O. Box 935
Harrow
HA1 3YJ
Patient line: 0181 423 8999
Provides a range of leaflets including 'Consent Matters', 'Access to Medical
Records' and 'Making the Most of Your Doctor'
http://www.pat-assoc.org/

People for the Ethical Treatment of Animals (PETA)
P.O. Box 3169
London
NW1 2JF

Pituitary Foundation
P.O. Box 1944
Bristol
BS99 2UB
Email: helpline@pitpat.demon.co.uk

Polycystic Ovarian Support Group (UK)
P.O. Box 4305
Great Barr
Birmingham
B42 2EL

Premature Menopause Group (NZ)
c/o Dr Andrew Shelling
Dept of Obstetrics and Gynaecology
National Women's Hospital
Claude Road
Auckland
New Zealand

Premature Menopause Support Group
P.O. Box 392
High Wycombe
HP15 7SH
http://www.daisychain.org/

Premature Ovarian Failure Support Group (USA)
P.O. Box 23643
Alexandria
Virginia 22304
USA
http://pofsupport.org/

Royal College of Obstetricians and Gynaecologists Bookshop
27 Sussex Place
Regent's Park
London
NW1 4RG
Publishes range of patient information.

Society of Homoeopaths
2 Artizan Road
Northampton
NN1 4HU
01602 21400

The Turner Syndrome Society
1/8 Irving Court
Hardgate
Clydebank
G81 6BA
01389 380385
http://www.tss.org.uk/

Turner's Syndrome Society of Canada
814 Glencairn Ave
Toronto
Ontario
M6B 2A3
Canada

Turner's Syndrome Society of the US
1313 Southeast 5th St
Suite 327
Minneapolis
Minnesota 55414
USA
http://www.turner-syndrome-us.org/

Verity
30 Chalton House
Chalton Street
London
NW1 1HH
Offers polycystic ovarian syndrome (PCOS) support.
See also http://www.pcosupport.org

Victorian Turner's Syndrome Association Inc.
31 Price St
Essendon
Victoria
Australia 3040

WellBeing (RCOG Health Research Charity for Women and Babies)
27 Sussex Place
Regent's Park
London
NW1 4SP
Royal College of Obstetricians and Gynaecologists charity which provides information for women and raises research funds.

What Doctors Don't Tell You Ltd
4 Wallace Road
London
N1 2PG

Women's Health (Resource and Information Centre)
52 Featherstone Street
London
EC1Y 8RT
Health enquiry line: 0171 251 6580
Library, newsletter and mail-order leaflets; can advise on nearest menopause clinic.

Women's Health Concern
P.O. Box 1629
London
W8 6AU
0171 938 3932

World Society for the Protection of Animals (WSPA)
2 Langley Lane
London
SW8 1TJ
0171 793 0540
Information on Premarin.

Further Internet information

General

Free access to Medline Plus	http://www.nlm.gov
Internet Overview of Women's Health	http://cpmcnet.columbia.edu/dept/rosenthal

Menopause

Menopaus List	http://www.howdyneighbor./com/menopaus/index.html
	http://www.oxford.net/~tishy/elists.html
	http://www.members.aol.com/Menochat
ASM	alt.support.meno

Surgical menopause

Sans-uteri	http://www.2cowherd.net/findings/sans-uteri.html
Witsendo	http://www.endometriosis.org/endowits.html
	alt.support.endo

GLOSSARY

Agenesis	Term used to mean lack of development or 'not coming into being'.
AIS	Androgen insensitivity syndrome, an intersex condition previously known as testicular feminization (TF) or male pseudohermaphroditism. Other earlier names include Morris's syndrome, Goldberg-Maxwell syndrome, Gilbert-Dreyfus syndrome, Rosewater syndrome, Lubs syndrome and Reinfenstein syndrome.
AMH	Anti-Müllerian hormone, also known as MIS (Müllerian inhibiting substance). *See* Müllerian ducts.
Androgens	Masculinizing hormones, e.g. testosterone.
Atresia	Term which means 'without an opening'; used medically to refer to lack of a vaginal opening (vaginal atresia) and follicles which do not open to release their eggs (atretic ovarian follicles).
CAH	Congenital adrenal hyperplasia, an intersex condition.
CAIS	'Complete' form of AIS.
Candida	Shorthand term for candida albicans, a yeast which can cause problems in the vagina and more generally.
CAT scan	Computerized axial tomography. Type of scan

	sometimes used to measure bone density, also referred to as QCT (qualitative computed tomography) scan.
'Chocolate' cyst	Medical term used to describe the thick dark contents of the blood-filled ovarian cysts which can develop with endometriosis, for instance. Also known as 'tarry' cyst.
Corpus luteum	Medical term for sac remaining after an ovarian follicle has burst; named after its appearance ('body yellow').
D&C	Abbreviation for 'dilatation and curettage', medical procedure to scrape away growth of the womb lining.
Dermoid	Medical term for a type of ovarian cyst.
DHT	Dihydrotestosterone; one of the androgen family of hormones.
Diuretics	Drugs used to treat water retention.
DXA	Dual energy X-ray absorptiometry, also abbreviated as DEXA. DXA machines measure bone mineral density.
Epidemiology	Study of patterns and possible causes of disease in the population at large rather than individuals.
'Female' duct system	Term used in this book for the Müllerian ducts, which have the capacity to develop into female organs. *See* Müllerian ducts.
FSH	Follicle-stimulating hormone released by the pituitary gland.
Genital cell cluster	Term used in this book for urogenital sinus. *See* urogenital sinus.

Germ cells	Medical term for cells that become eggs or sperm; simply described as future egg/sperm cells in this book.
Gestone	Intra-muscular injections of progesterone which can be used to support early stages of pregnancy after fertility treatment.
GIFT	Stands for gamete intra-Fallopian transfer; a less specialized form of fertility treatment than IVF, it involves mixing a few collected eggs with sperm and immediately transferring them into one of the Fallopian tubes (where conception occurs normally). Unlike IVF, embryos are not created outside the body first and then placed in the uterus. GIFT can be more acceptable to couples who have religious or ethical objections to IVF.
GnRH	Gonadotrophin-releasing hormone released by the hypothalamus to prompt the pituitary to release gonadotrophins (the collective term for hormones which affect the gonads, i.e. FSH and LH)
Gonadal dysgenesis	Lack of development of the gonads; also known as gonadal agenesis.
Gonadal ridge	Medical term for site in the embryo where ovaries or testes develop; simply described as 'long bundles' in this book.
Gonadectomy	Surgical removal of the gonads (see below); more specifically orchidectomy when removal of the testes.
Gonads	Collective term which can be used for ovaries or testes.

hCG	Human chorionic gonadotrophin; hormone produced by a fertilized egg to signal its presence to its mother's body and prevent menstruation. Also the hormone measured in pregnancy tests.
HDL	High-density lipoprotein; type of blood fat studied in relation to heart disease.
HRT	Hormone replacement therapy.
Intersex	Term used for medical conditions which lead to a person being born with male *and* female physical characteristics. Not to be confused with transsexual, where a person has male *or* female characteristics but wishes to change them.
IVF	In-vitro fertilization, also known as 'test-tube' fertilization.
Laparoscopy	Medical term for exploratory investigation that involves examining the abdominal organs through a minor incision using a special instrument called a laparoscope.
Laparotomy	Medical term for major abdominal operation; can be exploratory.
LDL	Low-density lipoprotein; type of blood fat studied in relation to heart disease.
Leaky gut	Term used to describe problems that are thought to develop when the lining of the gut becomes sensitive to certain foods and therefore allows larger food molecules to 'leak' into the body.
LH	Luteinizing hormone, released by the pituitary gland.

Long bundles	Term used in this book for the gonadal ridge in the embryo. *See* gonadal ridge.
'Male' duct system	Term used in this book for the Wolffian duct system, which has the capacity to develop into male organs. *See* Wolffian ducts.
MIS	Müllerian inhibiting substance, also known as AMH (anti-Müllerian hormone).
MPA	Medroxyprogesterone acetate; one of the progestogens.
MRI scan	Magnetic resonance imaging scan; specialized scan used to obtain high-quality pictures of areas such as the pituitary gland at the base of the brain.
MRKH syndrome	Mayer-Rokitansky-Kuster-Hauser syndrome; may also be referred to as vaginal agenesis.
Müllerian ducts	'Female' duct system in the embryo, also known as paramesonephric ducts; lack of development of these ducts can be referred to as Müllerian duct dysplasia or aplasia.
Oophorectomy	Surgical removal of one or both ovaries. The full medical term for removal of both ovaries and Fallopian tubes is bilateral salpingo-oophorectomy (BSO).
Orchidectomy	*See* gonadectomy.
PAIS	'Partial' form of AIS.
PCOS	Polycystic ovarian syndrome.
POF	Premature ovarian failure.
Primary hypogonadism	Lack of hormone secretion by the ovaries (or

	testes), e.g. due to ovarian failure, Turner syndrome, etc.
QCT	*See* CAT scan.
SD	Standard deviation; statistic measuring variation.
'Streak' ovaries	Thin streaks of white fibrous ovarian tissue instead of ovaries.
Sub-total hysterectomy	Hysterectomy in which the cervix is left in place.
TDF	Testes determining factor; supposed substance produced by part of the Y chromosome to stimulate the development of testes.
Testes	Two organs which house sperm; equivalent to the ovaries, which store eggs. The testes develop in the abdomen and then move into the testicles in boys and men.
TS	Turner syndrome; also known as Turner's syndrome.
Urogenital sinus	Medical term for part of the embryo that develops into the genitals and urinary outlet; simply described as genital cell cluster in this book.
Williams procedure	Type of plastic surgery to construct vagina.
Wolffian ducts	'Male' duct system in the embryo, also known as mesonephric ducts.
XX	Shorthand used for sex chromosome pair with two X chromosomes.
XY	Shorthand used for sex chromosome pair with an X and a Y chromosome.

Index

Page entries appearing in italics refer to figures.